DATE DUE

FEB 08 '80		
APR 04 '80		
GAYLORD		PRINTED IN U.S.A.

HEART CARE

Contributing Specialists

HEART CARE

AN AUTHORITATIVE GUIDE BY TWENTY EXPERTS

Edited by

Morris Fishbein, M.D.

Medical Editor
Britannica Book of the Year
Editor
Modern Home Medical Adviser
The Modern Family Health Guide

HANOVER HOUSE
Garden City, New York

DEDICATION

Dedicated to the Chicago Heart Association, with which the editor has been associated since 1924 when it was founded. All royalties derived from this book will be paid to the Chicago Heart Association, to be devoted to research on the heart.

Preface

Heart disease is the leading cause of death in the United States. No doubt heart disease will always be the leading cause of death as more and more diseases are conquered. All tissues eventually lose the power of growth and repair; when the heart stops beating, life ends.

During the last fifty years, increased knowledge of the heart has resulted in postponing death in hundreds of thousands of cases. In 1960 children born with congenitally deformed hearts can, in the vast majority of cases, be saved by newly developed surgical procedures, which are fully described in this book.

Rheumatic fever, which used to be the leading cause of death in children between five and fifteen, is beginning to yield to medical study and will probably be conquered in the not too distant future. Already several research institutions are approaching success with a vaccine, or immunizing technique, which can aid in the prevention of rheumatic fever in children.

Infectious conditions, such as those produced by the streptococci, which can infect the heart causing endocarditis, are being controlled by antibiotic drugs. Formerly, the condition called subacute bacterial endocarditis was invariably fatal.

As people grow older and are subjected to increasing stresses, including infections, overexertion, fatigue, and emotional strain, the heart begins to show changes which may seriously endanger life. Excessive action of the thyroid gland speeds up the heart. An excess of glandular material pouring into the blood may similarly interfere with the beat of the heart.

In this book leading authorities explain the methods by which modern medicine detects changes in the heart and the new methods of treatment that are available to block or overcome these menaces. Proof is already available that proper treatment with the new drugs, such as the tranquilizers and psychic energizers and those that can control the rate of the heartbeat and its intensity, may be important in prolonging life and restoring the heart to normal. New drugs have been developed which can eliminate excess fluid from the body, thus lessening the work of the heart. From all of this has come a personal hygiene of the heart which should be known to every person, particularly the elderly, and which may give them increased freedom from distress and may prolong their lives.

My great appreciation is due to the specialists in cardiology, the study of the heart, who have cooperated in preparing the articles for this volume and who have gladly elected that all royalties from the book will be devoted to heart research.

My special thanks are due to my wife, Anna Mantel Fishbein, who has read every word of every article, editing and revising, and whose suggestions have contributed so much to the readability and easy understanding of the book.

Morris Fishbein

Chicago
May 1960

CONTENTS

Contents

Introduction: The Prevention and Control of Heart Disease

MORRIS FISHBEIN, M.D.

THE HEART of a child at birth weighs less than an ounce. When the child becomes an adult, the heart weighs one-half pound. The stimulus for the heartbeat is in certain nervous tissue which is called the pacemaker of the heart. The amount of the energy developed has been calculated as 1/1000 volt. The heart of a child beats around 100 times a minute; the rate of the adult heart averages 72 times a minute.

Again and again you will read in these pages that the heart is a pump. It circulates blood through the body, moving 500 gallons of blood each day. The calculations indicate that the heart beats 2.5 billion times during the life of a human being, averaging seventy years. Remember that the heart begins to work before the child is born and is never quiet until death. When the heart rests, it can rest only by slowing the rate of the beat and by slightly decreasing its force. Thus this vital organ never gets a complete rest. For that reason our heart must be protected in every possible way against overwork and injury.

In the middle years of the twentieth century diseases of the heart and heart failure lead all other causes of death. Even if a disease of the heart or its failure does not result in death, it may result in long periods of incapacity and partial living.

For centuries the heart was considered the seat of the soul, the center of life. Therefore the heart was often associated with the idea of courage, as in the phrases "stout heart" or "faint heart." A man lacking initiative may be called "weakhearted" and a man of exceptional courage may be called "stronghearted." Moreover, the heart is so closely allied with emotions, particularly passion and love, that the word for heart in every language is sung again and again in the ballads and lyrics and arias of popular music and opera.

The heart is an involuntary muscle. Most of the muscles of the body can be moved as we will them to move. Perhaps only two or three instances are recorded in medical history of people who were able to control the heartbeat voluntarily. In fact, one instance is recorded in which a human being was able to stop his heartbeat temporarily.

HEREDITY AND HEART DISEASE

The main causes of congenital malformations of the heart and the large blood vessels are unusual influences that act through the mother, such as occur when the mother may have had German measles or other virus disorders early in her pregnancy; changes in the genes which are responsible for the type of the child; and interactions between the genetic and environmental factors that prevail in the mother and her prospective child. Modern medicine is in its very infancy as far as hereditary factors are concerned. The time may come when by chemical or physical methods changes in the tissues at their earliest stages may become effective.

ENVIRONMENTAL FACTORS

In a recent discussion of the prevention and control of heart disease held before the American Public Health Association, Dr. Irving S. Wright emphasized that overweight in itself is not a cause of heart disease or hardening of the arteries. In fact, complicated interrelationships of many factors are involved. These may include the total calories taken in, the total amount of fat, the saturated fats as compared with the unsaturated fats, the amount of cholesterol, and other factors related to the glands of internal secretion. People who smoke excessively seem to have higher blood pressures, but people who smoke excessively may also be people who lead lives of higher stress and tension. Dr. Wright notes that they are the men who frequently eat too much, drink too much, sleep too light, work too hard, and get themselves into all kinds of stressful situations. "These are the men," he says, "who argue about an extra egg on their hotel bill and who become red-faced and irritated about matters of little consequence in terms of health."

Dr. Wright has noted people who have the capacity to tolerate high blood pressure. He notes a woman who has been a great grandmother four times and who for thirty-five years has had a blood pressure of 240 when the heart contracts and 130 when the heart is relaxed. This woman had never had a stroke or a heart attack. She had been unable to get blood pressure lowering effects with the new drugs, which apparently disagreed with her.

Dr. Wright has offered special encouragement to people who have coronary attacks or myocardial infarctions. Many of these attacks are unrecognized. At post-mortem examinations we see great numbers of bodies in which the heart carries the relics of previous heart attacks which appear as scars in the heart muscle. Dr. Wright finds that only from 10 to 15 per cent of people with blocking of the blood vessels of the heart die rather suddenly, and he believes that with the modern anticoagulant drugs the rate will come down even to 5 per cent.

THE ANTICOAGULANT DRUGS

The evidence is clear that the death rate from clots in the heart or clots in the blood vessels of the brain are greatly lessened by the use of the new anticoagulant drugs. The number of deaths has been reduced by one-third and the complications from such clots by approximately four-fifths. In an extensive study made in Great Britain, investigators found that men under fifty-five years of age who had initial attacks of blocking of the coronary blood vessels of the heart had recurrences only one-fifth as often when anticoagulant drugs were used as when they were not used. In men over the age of fifty-five the recurrences were reduced by one-half. This is a most encouraging outlook.

THE OUTLOOK

There are three groups of heart conditions in which definite progress can be made. Rheumatic fever is now being greatly reduced in incidence by the prompt treatment of serious infections of the throat. For the control of the streptococcus that is associated with rheumatic fever, the sulfonamide drugs and the antibiotics bring about destruction of the germs and thereby the attack on the heart by the poisonous products that come from the streptococcus. Rheumatic fever was once the leading cause of death of children aged five to fifteen but now the number of such cases has been greatly reduced. Accidents have superseded rheumatic fever as the leading cause of death in young children.

The second great problem in heart disease is the death of people of advancing years who suffer from failure of this vital organ. People live much longer than they used to live. The diseases that involve breakdown of the heart affect men far more than they do women. Physicians associate the increased number of deaths related to the heart which occur in men to the fact that men are more greatly exposed to overwork, to stress and strain, and to obnoxious factors in the environment than are women.

The third group of heart conditions are those affecting old people who begin to suffer with inflammations of the various tissues of the body and with breakdown. Through proper study of such cases and through the development of better hospital services for older people, the rate of heart failure in older people will definitely be lowered.

Primary in the treatment of all types of conditions affecting the heart is adequate rest. With rest must come also relaxation. The number of beds available in hospitals and institutions in the United States for people with heart disease is far below the number actually required. Moreover, rehabilitation is possible for older people with heart disease. This involves adequate diet with proper hormones and vitamins and minerals as well as proper amounts of protein. Furthermore, all of our authorities emphasize the necessity for a certain amount of controlled exercise as well as for rest. The basic factor in living human tissues is the importance of use. Pathologists recognize what they call atrophy of disuse. In other words, failure to use the tissues results in their breakdown.

A FORMULA FOR AGING

People who live long usually have five factors in their bodies which are lower than the average. These are 1) a low diet, 2) a low blood pressure, 3) a low pulse rate, 4) a low basal metabolism, and 5) a low threshold for the sense of humor. People who laugh easily are likely to avoid stress.

People who have had coronary thrombosis or blocking of the blood vessels of the heart need to learn to live at a somewhat slower pace. They must plan a definite schedule of relaxed living and select a rest period during each day, which must be positively observed. Dr. George R. Herrmann suggests that they begin the day with breakfast in bed between 8 and 9 o'clock in the morning, rest a half-hour afterward while reading the papers, and then leisurely get up, shave, and dress. Any work that is to be done should be approached without hurry or excessive emotion.

Mental hygiene is essentially a technique of practicing living without worry. There are innumerable aphorisms—such as "Tomorrow is another day"—which indicate that the problems of the moment tend to solve themselves if given a little extra time.

Many ways of relaxing are known to all of us, but even hobbies may be pursued with stress. A golfer must learn to use a cart if that is available, to stop at six, nine, or any other number of holes when he feels that he has had enough. People who play cards for relaxation should keep the stakes so low that the strain of excessive losses will not disturb them. Even people who walk should choose walks on level ground and should pace themselves so that the walking does not lead to exhaustion.

At work, periods may be taken after one, two, or three hours of work for relaxation. The important executive should not hesitate to have a couch in the office on which he may recline for brief periods. In the absence of the ability to recline, one may still remain quietly at the desk. Sometimes an executive is surrounded with assistants, secretaries, or other personnel who are themselves subject to worrying, pushing, striving, and stress. An executive who wants to practice good mental hygiene should have people around him who aid his tranquillity and who do not disturb his equanimity.

Most of the hours of our days are spent in attending to our own wants. Learn to do these things without stress or strain. The elimination should be done when the urge comes and not postponed and should be given sufficient time to avoid straining. Eating should be done under leisurely conditions, in pleasant surroundings and congenial atmosphere, and not when the person is tense or tired. Business conferences during meals should be avoided. A light breakfast and light dinner with a rather heavier lunch is preferable to a heavy dinner late at night. The person with coronary attacks should avoid banquets. Most nutritionists suggest five small meals daily rather than three heavier ones.

Tea and coffee contain caffeine which is a stimulant drug. Persons who are avoiding stimulation should limit coffee and tea to a half-cup at breakfast and dinner but should avoid even this amount if it tends to produce sleeplessness or nervousness.

The man or woman who has had a coronary attack is advised to avoid crowds, gatherings at clubs, race tracks, or any situation in which noise and confusion predominate. The experts advise a person who has had a coronary attack to avoid campaigns or holding of any kind of public office; the civic duties must be left to those who are better able to perform them.

The life of the coronary invalid is a life of restriction, but the restrictions may be so planned as to make life still much worth living. One avoids climbing too many stairs. One avoids dances that require too much speed in motion. Sudden starts and heavy lifting are dangerous. Driving an automobile in heavy traffic and parking are frequently devastating. Walking is the best exercise. Fishing is the best recreation, solitaire the best card game. And above all of these music as a means of relaxation is encouraged.

Even books can be used as therapy. Travel books, biographies, and historical novels are relaxing. Mysteries, detective stories, erotic works, sex stimulants, and shocking writings must certainly be discouraged.

CHAPTER I

The Normal Heart

PAUL DUDLEY WHITE, M.D.

THE RANGE of the normal characteristics of the human heart is so great that its limits have not, even yet, been adequately explored. Considerable danger is always present of labeling as abnormal, as evidence of heart disease, variations from the normal that are simply unusual or rarely seen. Since more is probably now known about the diseased heart than about the normal one, an obscure symptom or observation not definitely known to be a manifestation of heart disease is something merely to follow up at intervals without any immediate commitment to serious interpretation.

A tall, slender, nervous woman will have a much smaller, more vertical, faster heart than a short, heavy, stolid man. Normal people of the same sex, age, and body build, especially of the same weight and height, may have hearts quite different in size and shape. Their pulse rate, blood pressure, electrocardiogram, and chest X-ray picture may be quite different. Here heredity plays a considerable role. For example, identical twins resemble each other closely in these various characteristics, but they are not identical for each. To establish each individual's own norm, each young adult while still in good health should obtain and preserve in his own file for future reference his pulse rate at rest, blood pressure, electrocardiogram, and chest X ray. In 1707, Sir John Floyer, the physician who first used a watch to count the pulse, recommended such a recording of the pulse rate. Individual records of these basic data ought to be made also because current tables relating these to age, sex, height, and weight are inadequate.

THE AVERAGE FINDINGS

The heart is primarily a muscular pump comprised of extremely efficient and powerful, although not very large, spiral and circular bands of specialized muscle fibers. In their contraction, these muscle fibers squeeze the blood out of the two (left and right) ventricular chambers into the aorta and pulmonary artery respectively. During this process a shortening of the longitudinal axis of the heart occurs from base to apex, both of which are involved.

The muscle of the left ventricle of the heart weighs nearly twice as much as the muscle of the right ventricle—130 grams (or about 4.06 ounces) compared with 70 grams (or about 2.19 ounces), in the average human adult. The muscle of the left ventricle, moreover, has much more work to do, in pumping blood all over the body, than the muscle of the right ventricle, which pumps blood through the lungs. The capacities of the two ventricles are about equal—130 milliliters or cubic centimeters (about 4.4 fluid ounces). About the same amount of blood must be pumped out of each ventricle with each heartbeat—approximately 50 to 100 milliliters at rest (1.7 to 3.4 fluid ounces)—in order to avoid an excess of blood in the lungs or in the systemic circulation. The two ventricles are closely joined in their muscular structure, but their cavities are separated by a muscular septum or partition of muscular tissue, which develops during the fetal period.

In addition to these two pumping chambers or ventricles, the heart has two other chambers, the right and left atria. These thin-walled, distensible muscular cavities are receiving chambers for the ventricles. The right atrium receives the venous or "blue" blood from the head, arms, abdomen, and legs through the great veins called the superior and inferior venae cavae, while the left atrium receives the oxygenated or "red" blood from the lungs by way of the pulmonary veins.

Other vital parts of the pumping mechanism are the valves, of which there are four. Two valves separate the two atria from the two ventricles to prevent a return of blood to the atria when the ventricles contract. The one on the left side is called the mitral valve: like a bishop's miter, it has two sides or cusps or is bicuspid. The valve separating the right ventricle from the right atrium is called the tricuspid because it has three sides or leaves. The other two valves are also tricuspid, but the one on the left side is called the aortic valve. This valve prevents a reflux or regurgitation of blood from the aorta into the left ventricle when that ventricle relaxes (or is in diastole) to get ready for the next beat or contraction (systole). The valve on the right side, called the pulmonic valve, protects the right ventricular cavity from blood that would otherwise regurgitate from the pulmonary artery.

The heartbeat starts automatically from a small structure of nerve and muscle called the pacemaker or sinoatrial node, which is located at the junction of the superior vena cava and the right atrium. The beat travels electrically and mechanically in a continuous, or peristaltic, wave over the thin atrial muscular wall to another specialized neuromuscular structure called the atrioventricular node, or nerve center for the ventricle. These nodes or nerve centers are so small that they

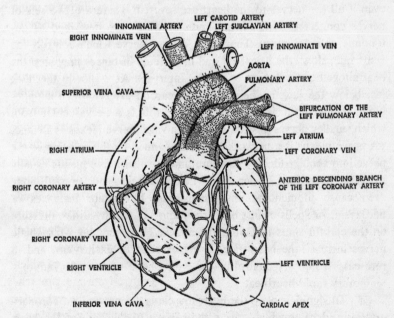

Front View of the Heart, Showing the Principal Structures.

Illustration courtesy Denoyer-Geppert Company

can be seen only under the microscope. From the atrioventricular node the heartbeat travels on, at an accelerated rate of a meter (39.3 inches) per second, through a special muscle bundle and its branches into both ventricles where it ends in multitudinous contracting muscle fibers to initiate the ventricular beat. Normally, an interval of a little less than one-fifth of a second elapses between the onset of the atrial contraction, represented by the so-called P wave of the electrocardiogram, and the onset of the ventricular contraction, represented by the QRS wave. The duration of the ventricular contraction or systole, from the onset of the QRS wave to the end of the T wave, is normally one-third of a second in the case of a human heart at a rate of 60 beats per minute. This means that the resting period of the ventricles or diastole lasts two-thirds of a second, which at this heart rate comprises an eight-hour day of work.

Nerve connections to the heart are of great significance, although the heart can continue to beat, because of its automatic pacemaker, even if all the nerves to the heart are severed. There are two sets of nerves connected to the heart, both of which are described as autonomic or involuntary. The vagus, a large nerve which controls the heart rate, slows the heartbeat and in extreme instances may stop the beat altogether for longer or shorter intervals. At a spot in the neck just below the jaw, in the wall of the carotid artery, which supplies blood to the brain, is the carotid sinus: this is a nerve center from which smaller nerves pass on and here a vagal nerve plexus is located. (A nerve plexus is a network of nerves formed by the splitting of the nerve into smaller fibers.) Pressure on the vagal nerve plexus usually slows the heart rate. Under unusual circumstances such pressure may even cause momentary unconsciousness. In certain instances of paroxysms or spells of fast heart rate, known as tachycardia, pressure on the carotid sinus may stop the attack. However, the sympathetic nerves increase the heart rate during exercise or excitement, and in rare cases voluntary control of the sympathetic nerves may induce a temporary rapid heartbeat.

Of vital significance to the heart muscle is the network of coronary arteries and veins which covers the surface of the base of the heart like a crown (Latin, *corona*). Two main arterial trunks (left and right), given off by the aorta just above the aortic valve, bring fresh arterial blood during early diastole to the heart muscle. The left artery is usually much the larger and divides quickly into two branches, the circumflex and the anterior descending branches. The latter, quite important, is sometimes called "the artery of sudden death," since a clot or thrombus near its mouth is a common occurrence in the case of a serious heart attack. A considerable interlacing or anastomosis of the smallest twigs of the various branches of the coronary tree, under increasing pressure and demands later in life due to atherosclerotic narrowing of the major coronary arterial trunks, may act as a collateral circulation to by-pass points of severe narrowing and block, and thereby saves lives. The coronary veins collect the blood that has oxygenated and nourished the heart muscle to return it through the coronary sinus to the right atrial chamber where other blue blood enters from the two venae cavae.

Lining the inside of the four heart chambers and the surface of the valves is the endocardium, a delicate membrane which may be injured by infection, as in endocarditis, or by the deposition of a clot, or thrombosis. On the outside of the heart is another membrane called the pericardium, which protects and lubricates it in the so-called pericardial sac. This too may be infected, as in pericarditis, or, it may be scarred or infarcted by the cutting-off of its blood supply. When infected or otherwise injured, the sac may be filled with an effusion of fluid or even with blood.

The heart as a pump is the mainspring of the circulation, and it is greatly aided by accessory structures, the integrity of which is of much importance. For example:

a) Elasticity of the aorta and its main branches. Loss of this elasticity with age and/or disease reduces the efficiency of the circulation and places more demands on the heart.

b) The muscular activity of the arterioles which divert the blood to those areas of the body where it is temporarily most needed.

c) The valves in the veins, especially of the legs, which help to direct the blood in the proper way. When defective, postural stasis and hypotension of serious degree may occur.

d) Good muscle tone in the extremities, particularly of the legs. This in itself helps to pump blood back to the heart.

e) Free and vigorous motion of the diaphragm which, when in good tone, acts as part of an effective suction pump to bring both air and blood into the thorax.

Consider now the range of the normal heart and circulation, anatomically and physiologically, as examined in the clinic, doctor's office, or elsewhere. Again, every person reaching maturity should establish his own normal range for future use, since the difference from the "average" normal may be considerable.

SIZE AND WEIGHT OF THE HEART

The size and thereby the weight of the heart can be roughly estimated on physical examination but accurately measured only by X-ray study, either in the form of an X-ray film or visually by fluoroscopy. The size of the heart is usually said to vary according to the size of the person's two fists fitted together. This is generally true, but the actual volume varies between systole or ventricular contraction and diastole or ventricular dilatation, and again according to the heart rate. The faster the rate, the smaller is the heart volume in diastole. With an extremely slow rate of 40 to 45 beats per minute, which is not uncommon in trained athletes, definite variation in volume between systole and diastole occurs. A doubling of the output per beat develops, from about 60 milliliters or cubic centimeters (about 2 ounces) to 120 milliliters (about 4 ounces) for each ventricle. The volume of the human adult heart partially filled averages about 600 milliliters (about 1¼ pints).

The weight of the normal adult human heart varies from about 200 grams (7 ounces) in a very small woman to 350 grams (12 ounces) in a very large man. It equals slightly over 0.4 per cent of the total body weight. Thus a woman weighing 100 pounds should have a heart weighing a little less than ½ pound (about 220 grams), and a man weighing 200 pounds should have a heart weighing not quite ¾ pound (about 360 grams). We include in this weight the fat on the surface of the heart, or the visceral pericardium, and the first few centimeters of the great arteries and veins. At birth the heart weighs 20 to 25 grams or slightly less than one ounce; at one year 30 to 40, at four years 65 to 75, and at eight years 95 to 105 grams.

The length of the adult heart varies from 10 to 12 centimeters, averaging 11 (about 4.33 inches); the breadth ranges from 8 to 10 centimeters, averaging 9 (about 3.5 inches), and the depth from 6 to 8 centimeters, averaging 7 (about 2.75 inches).

As with the volume and weight of the heart, great variations in the position of the heart are observed in normal people. Position is dependent on the individual's height and weight but particularly on the shape of the thorax. Ordinarily, the taller the person, the more vertical is the heart position, due to a relatively low position of the diaphragm. In a short, stocky person with a high diaphragm, the heart lies much more horizontally. The more vertical the heart, the smaller it appears to be in the X-ray picture; the more horizontal it is, the larger its shadow. The shape of the thorax is, however, not always in accord with the height and weight of the individual. The longer the thorax, the more vertical the heart; the shorter the thorax, the more horizontal the heart. In some extreme cases, the heart shadow is scarcely visible behind the sternum, when the chest is long with a low diaphragm and the heart shadow is as much to the right as to the left. In many people body weight increases with age, and a slow elevation of the diaphragm results. Thus, in a period of fifteen to twenty years, the heart position may change from almost vertical to approximately horizontal. This change in position has a significant effect not only on the X-ray picture but also on the electrocardiogram, which may show a normal change of axis deviation from so-called right to so-called left.

Along with changes in position noted between vertical and horizontal, the physician notes the rotation of the heart. In a vertical heart, the left ventricle tends to be more completely posterior in position, with the right ventricle making up the anterior surface. When the heart is horizontal, a moderate amount of the left ventricle appears at the left border and may form a considerable part of the anterior surface. The left atrium is always posterior and the right atrium makes up part of the anterior surface of the heart and the right border. Lack of

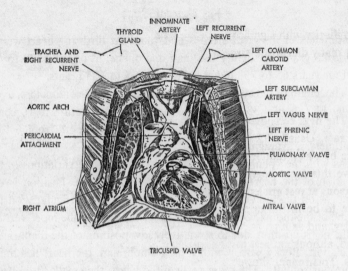

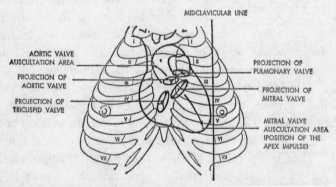

Relative positions of the heart and the blood vessels connected with it, along with important structures within the heart, are shown in the top drawing; the heart chambers and vessels are represented in a distended or expanded state.

Normal position of the heart within the rib cage is shown in the diagram. The two *auscultation areas* are the principal locations from which the heart sounds are heard. The physician can usually determine the position of the heart by palpation, or feeling with the hands on the surface of the body, and auscultation, or detecting and interpreting the heart sounds. First step is locating the cardiac apex; it should lie between the fifth and sixth left ribs on or just to the right of the *midclavicular line,* which is a vertical line dropped from a point halfway between the middle of the breastbone and the outer end of the left collarbone. The maximal impulse or beat in this auscultation area identifies the site of the cardiac apex.

(From Heart Disease, *4th Edition, by Paul Dudley White, M.D., copyright 1951. Used by permission of the publishers, The Macmillan Company.)*

familiarity with significant variations of position of the heart accounts for many diagnostic errors.

THE HEART RATE

The next consideration in the range of the normal heart is that of its rate. Usually 72 beats per minute is considered the normal pulse rate but, as a matter of fact, only a small minority of people actually have this exact heart rate. The extremes of rate in perfectly normal persons at rest are extraordinary. I myself have found the resting heart rate to be in the upper 30s per minute in a well-trained champion miler, and as high as 118 per minute in a champion marathon runner who, although at rest just before the start of the race, was highly nervous. This runner showed a rate of 108, ten beats slower, after running twenty-six miles and winning the race with ease.

Variation in heart rate may develop in any person, depending on many factors. In the early morning before the person gets started for the day, his pulse tends to be at its slowest. Many people with heart rates in the upper 40s or 50s in the morning may have pulse rates in the 80s at the end of a busy day. Exercise, excitement, fatigue, infection, and various diseases can elevate the heart rate noticeably, while tobacco, coffee, tea, and alcohol may also increase the rate in many people. Rest as in sleep, cold, and carotid sinus pressure (pressure over the carotid artery in the neck) decrease the heart rate.

A few persons have been recorded who can voluntarily accelerate their heart rates. In two instances, which I myself studied and reported many years ago, heart rates almost doubled (from 90 to 160) for a few seconds to a few minutes without any change except the will of the person to produce a fast pulse. One person, but only one that I have heard about, has been cited as being able to slow his heart rate voluntarily. The voluntary control of the vagus nerve is undoubtedly a much rarer phenomenon than control of the sympathetic nerves.

At birth the heart rate averages 130 to 140, slightly faster in girls than in boys, and the rate slowly decreases until it drops below 100 at rest at about five or six years of age.

HEART RHYTHM

The rhythm of the heart is usually regular but often disturbed rhythm, called sinus arrhythmia, occurs because of a variation in the rate at which the electrical impulses are sent out from the pacemaker or sinoatrial node previously described. Sinus arrhythmia is common in normal children and young adults and has been seen also in a few very old people. The rhythm is noticeably increased with respiration. During deep inspiration the pulse quickens and during full expiration it slows, particularly toward the end of each respiratory movement. This definite change in rhythm may in a few cases be extreme, amounting sometimes to as much as 30 or more beats per minute, leaving the rate at 45 to 50 beats in deep expiration and 80 to 85 in full inspiration.

Other disturbances of rhythm can occur in normal hearts: for example, premature beats, sometimes called extrasystoles. These are normally common but they may be disturbing to the person who experiences them. In the absence of any other evidence of trouble, they are quite harmless and are simply indicative of an excessive temporary irritability of some part of the heart muscle other than the pacemaker. Arrhythmia, it must be remembered, can also be produced by disease, but the great majority of persons who show extrasystoles or premature beats do have healthy hearts. Tobacco and various other toxic and stimulating factors can easily induce extrasystoles in susceptible persons. When extrasystoles come in rapid succession they can produce paroxysmal tachycardia, or even paroxysmal flutter or fibrillation, although the latter are more common in the presence of heart disease than in normal hearts. Such paroxysms of tachycardia of one kind or another can be distressing. They are, however, usually relatively insignificant, and if the heart is otherwise normal, they are not harmful. Often these symptoms can be controlled by omitting excessive stimuli such as those from tobacco or by taking medicines such as quinidine or mild sedatives.

BLOOD PRESSURE

The blood pressure also varies greatly from one healthy person to another. In infancy the blood pressure may be quite low; for example, 80 systolic and 50 to 60 diastolic. In childhood the blood pressure approaches 100 systolic and 70 diastolic. In adult life the normal range is considerable, from 100 to 150 systolic and from 60 to 90 diastolic. Everyone should know his usual blood pressure. For a person whose blood pressure is usually low, about 105 systolic, a pressure of 150 or 155 is an elevation. However, in every individual a diurnal variation occurs. In the morning before arising, the pressure may be as low as 110 systolic and 70 diastolic, and at the end of a busy day it may have risen to 140 systolic and 90 diastolic. The same factors that raise the heart rate tend to heighten the blood pressure. Exercise, excitement, and tobacco increase the pressure ordinarily, but some of the factors causing tachycardia or rapid heartbeat, such as fever and infection, do not increase the blood pressure; they may actually cause a decline in pressure.

HEART SOUNDS

The heart sounds, heard by auscultation, also vary greatly from person to person. The first sound is caused chiefly by closure of the mitral and tricuspid valves at the beginning of the contraction of the two ventricles. The second sound is produced by closure of the aortic and pulmonary valves at the end of that contraction, or systole. Sometimes early in diastole a faint third sound, heard normally, is much accentuated, producing a so-called gallop rhythm when the ventricular cavities are greatly dilated and the muscle is weak. Heart sounds are easily heard with the ear applied to the chest in almost all persons, but if the chest wall is thick or the lungs expanded, as in asthma with emphysema, the sounds may be distant and exceedingly decreased even though the heart is normal. In persons with thin chest walls, the sounds may be unusually loud. Many persons have reduplication, or the doubling of one sound or the other normally. This condition is due to asynchronous closure of the mitral and tricuspid valves in the case of the first sound, and similarly with the aortic and pulmonary valves when the second sound is doubled. Frequently both sounds are doubled normally. Exercise tends to increase the sounds while rest and sedatives decrease them.

Murmurs are due to vibrations of the walls of heart valves or blood vessels through which the blood is rushing when a variation in the caliber of the channel occurs. For example, there may be a narrowing of the valve or a leak; or an obstruction or an aneurysmal dilation may develop in the blood vessels.

Even heart murmurs may be normal. It is surprising that every normal person does not show them more readily because of the rush of blood through the heart chambers and into the great arteries. I myself can produce a systolic murmur in the pulmonary valve area in any normal person (more readily in a child) by the process of moderate exercise and then auscultation in the supine position, especially over the pulmonary valve area, where a slight-to-moderate systolic murmur can be easily heard. Almost all loud murmurs are, however, abnormal.

Earlier in this chapter I spoke of the importance of a normal young person keeping his electrocardiogram and chest X-ray film for future reference. The electrocardiogram is particularly valuable for a young male, because of the frequency with which coronary heart disease now occurs in the United States. Chest pain, whether or not due to coronary insufficiency, is a common symptom. When the electrocardiogram is taken, variations from the usual may arouse suspicion of the heart as a causative factor. In such cases comparison of the new electrocardiogram in all its details with that taken some months or years before, prior to the development of any chest pain, is most significant. Many times I have found it necessary to change the diagnosis in a young person from definite or possible "coronary heart disease" to "normal heart with a normal variation of certain complexes in the electrocardiogram." This has helped to dispel serious apprehension and a cardiac neurosis that was based on faulty interpretation of the electrocardiogram. Many factors, such as excitement, tobacco, position, and medicines, can change the electrocardiogram in the case of a normal

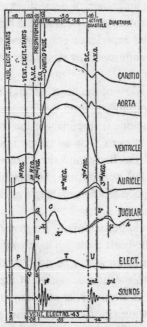

Chart shows the time relations of the electrocardiogram, atrial and ventricular contractions, pressure changes, and heart sounds. The electrocardiogram (second line from bottom) measures the electrical activity occurring during the heartbeat. The heartbeat goes from the sinoatrial node (in the right atrium) to the atrioventricular node and thence into the ventricles. Normally, an interval of a little less than a fifth of a second elapses between the beginning of the atrial contraction, called the P wave on the electrocardiogram, and the beginning of the ventricular contraction (see QRS on the electrocardiogram line, above). The duration of the ventricular contraction, represented by T on the electrocardiogram, is usually one-third of a second, at the heart rate of 60 beats per minute. The heart sounds, *1st* and *2nd* on the bottom line of the chart, are caused by the closing of the valves at the beginning of the ventricular contraction and at its ending.

(*From* The Mechanism and Graphic Registration of the Heart Beat, *by Sir Thomas Lewis, 1925, by permission of Shaw & Sons Ltd.*)

heart. Years ago in New York City some doctors, lawyers, insurance agents, and clients conspired to defraud insurance companies of millions of dollars by the simulation of heart disease in the electrocardiogram, by the administration of toxic doses of digitalis. This treachery was uncovered, and the experience emphasized that the normal electrocardiogram can be influenced by drugs and other elements as well as by disease.

As for the X-ray shadow of the heart, enough has been said already to indicate its great variability from one normal person to another, depending on many factors. These include the shape of the chest and other inherited tendencies as well as temporary conditions, such as heart rate, position of the body, and the amount of fat covering the outside of the heart and pericardium. Errors in interpretation have resulted from the presence of a large triangle of fat at the cardiac apex in especially obese persons.

Finally, a word should be said about heart symptoms in individuals with normal hearts. The heart itself is a highly sensitive structure nervously, and its vigorous beating may be unduly felt by susceptible persons. Palpitation, which means a sensation of the beating of the heart —slow or fast, regular or irregular, is common in normal persons and does not of itself indicate heart disease. Many normal persons who are unduly sensitive, perhaps nervously exhausted, have heartache over the heart itself, often with some local tenderness; in addition, they may note some disorder of breathing, particularly in the form of sighing dyspnea or shortness of breath. Such a person tends to feel faint easily and may actually lose consciousness occasionally. The combination of all these symptoms is called neurocirculatory asthenia, but *not* heart disease. During the First World War this condition was called soldier's heart or the effort syndrome. Most persons with this unusual sensitivity have normal hearts but are unduly worried about them. Actually, such people live longer than the average, being obliged to avoid extreme excesses of strain, tobacco, and alcohol because of these symptoms.

The true symptoms of heart disease are quite different. They include angina pectoris, which will be discussed later in the book, and shortness of breath due to congestion of the lungs. Swelling of the legs, sometimes a true symptom of heart disease, is more often the result of other causes, including the tendency of the local circulation to be obstructed in the veins. Overweight people who must stand for particularly long periods may have edema or swelling of legs that is produced simply by hydrostatic pressure in the upright position.

The heart and the other parts of the circulatory system form an extraordinary mechanism adapted to rapid changes of environmental factors. The heart is, as yet, impossible of duplication by any machine, although remarkable progress is being made in simulating the circulatory system (for short periods of time) by devices like the pump oxygenator. If no disease is present, the heart muscle does not ever actually wear out. It becomes less efficient in extreme old age, but some specific disease always ends life, whether or not it directly involves the heart.

CHAPTER II

Congenital Cardiac Defects

THOMAS J. DRY, M.B., Ch.B.

A "BLUE BABY" is a child born with an improperly formed heart or
congenital cardiac defect. But all children born with a congenital cardiac defect are not "blue." The ones who are blue have a defect that
permits venous or unoxygenated blood to mix with arterial or oxygenated blood.

Some babies have hearts so badly malformed that they die at birth
or soon afterwards. Others, less seriously handicapped, live longer—
perhaps to adult life and occasionally to advanced age. In general,
however, their life expectancy is shortened unless the defect can be
corrected by cardiac surgery.

Heart operations are now being performed all over the world, and
this has been possible just since 1940. At first, operations were done
only for defects outside the heart itself. It was early appreciated, however, that congenital heart defects within the heart might be operated
on only if some kind of pump mechanism could be developed that
could do the work of the heart and lungs, while the surgeon opened
the heart and corrected the defect.

The interest of research workers, who included scientists in many
fields besides heart specialists and surgeons, was aroused in many parts
of the world, and today the so-called heart-lung oxygenator is a reality. During the early work, another person, usually the father of the
patient, was used as a heart-lung machine. Naturally, this involved the
lives and health of two people, and the method was abandoned when
a satisfactory machine was devised. The development of the machines
and operations are described more fully in the chapter by Dr. Potts.

Dr. Paul Dudley White, in the first chapter, has described the normal heart, but to make clear the nature of the various individual congenital cardiac defects, some of the features of the normal heart must be emphasized again.

We speak and think of the heart as a single organ, yet in reality there are two hearts in this composite unit (see diagram on page 25). First, the right heart, meaning the right atrium and right ventricle, receives impure blood from all parts of the body and pumps it through the pulmonary artery and its branches into the lungs, where the impure blood becomes saturated with oxygen. Second, the left heart, left atrium and left ventricle, receives this purified blood from the pulmonary veins and pumps it through the aorta and its branches to all parts of the body. Therefore, although the right and left atria lie side by side and although the right and left ventricles are in a similar position, the lungs are interposed between the two hearts, so to speak. Furthermore, in the normal heart each of these sets of heart chambers is completely separated by a solid wall called a septum, the atrial septum (3, diagram) and the ventricular septum (6, diagram).

Another feature of the circulation which must be appreciated is that the pressure, built up when the left chambers contract and especially when the left ventricle contracts, is much higher than that built up by the right side of the heart. Actually the figures for the left and right ventricles are 120 and 20 millimeters of mercury respectively. This means that whenever an abnormal communication exists between any of the chambers of the heart, blood will flow from the left side of the heart to the right side with each heartbeat. Likewise, this will occur also if an abnormal communication exists between the aorta and the pulmonary artery: with each heartbeat, the blood will flow from the left to the right side of the heart.

Some tests have been devised which, though intricate and complicated, are extremely helpful in making an accurate diagnosis of congenital cardiac defects and aid in finding out whether or not any complications of the defect have occurred. In some instances the diagnosis can be made by ordinary office methods of examination. The physician can determine the extent of damage, if any, simply from what he sees with his eyes, what he feels with his hands, what he hears

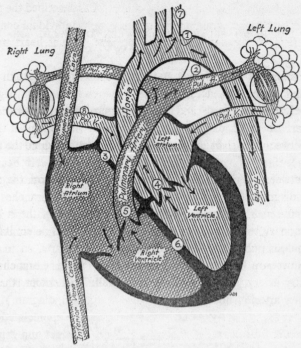

Diagram showing normal circulation of the blood through the heart, with the sites of the various congenital cardiac defects: 1) coarctation of the aorta; 2) ductus arteriosus: during intra-uterine life it conveys blood from the pulmonary artery to the aorta, after birth gradually shrinks and becomes a solid cord—if it does not, blood flows from the aorta to the pulmonary artery; 3) atrial septum, site of atrial septal defect; 4) aortic valve, site of aortic stenosis; 5) pulmonary valve, site of pulmonic stenosis; 6) ventricular septum, site of ventricular septal defect; 7) left subclavian artery which goes to the left arm; 8) one of the pulmonary veins.

through his stethoscope, and what is revealed to him by X ray and electrocardiograph. Occasionally, he doesn't even require an X-ray picture or an electrocardiogram.

Three varieties of these congenital cardiac defects are classified: a) an imperfect separation between the right and left hearts, so that the pure and impure bloods are mixed with one another; b) a narrowing in the path of flow of blood which causes an obstruction to the free flow of blood through the area; c) a combination of these two types of defects.

Separation between the left and right hearts can be incomplete in
any of five important places:

1) between the aorta and the pulmonary artery, called patent
ductus arteriosus (2, diagram).

2) between the right and left atria, called atrial septal defect (3,
diagram).

3) between the right and left ventricles, called ventricular septal defect (6, diagram).

4) between a pulmonary vein and the right side of the heart—all
the pulmonary veins should enter the left atrium. This defect is known
as anomalous pulmonary venous drainage.

5) between a branch of the pulmonary vein and a branch of the
pulmonary artery, that is, within a lung itself. This defect is called a
pulmonary arteriovenous fistula.

PATENT DUCTUS ARTERIOSUS

A patent ductus arteriosus, to repeat, is an abnormal connection
between the aorta and the pulmonary artery. The communication here,
however, is not caused by faulty development but is due to the lack of
closure of a blood vessel that connects the aorta and the pulmonary
artery. This blood vessel, the ductus arteriosus, has the special function, during intra-uterine life, of diverting the blood pumped out by
the right ventricle away from the pulmonary artery and into the aorta.
Obviously, circulation of blood through the lungs that will not function until the child draws its first breath would be superfluous. As soon
as the lungs do begin to function, the ductus automatically begins to
shrink; then all that remains of the ductus is a solid cord. Occasionally
this does not occur and the ductus remains open, or patent, hence
the name patent ductus arteriosus.

How does this handicap the circulation? With every heartbeat, from
20 to 75 per cent of the blood pumped out by the left ventricle escapes

from the aorta through the patent ductus into the pulmonary artery. This blood then must circulate through the lungs a second time. The left ventricle must then do an enormous amount of extra work in order to supply the amount of blood required by the body for its normal functions. Such an overworked left ventricle will enlarge and eventually result in heart failure.

At first the extra blood which passes through the lungs does not cause any trouble, since the lungs can accommodate a large amount of extra blood. In some cases, however, this tends to a narrowing of the small blood vessels in the lungs, and as this process continues the right ventricle must use increased force to pump the blood through the lungs and eventually it also is overworked. A direct consequence of these changes in the blood vessels in the lungs is a rise in the pressure in the right ventricle and in the pulmonary arteries. Eventually this pressure exceeds the pressure in the aorta, and as a result the impure blood from the pulmonary artery begins to flow through the patent ductus to mix with the pure blood in the aorta, and the patient becomes blue or cyanotic. Fortunately, physicians usually diagnose this condition early in life, advise surgical treatment, and so avoid the serious complication of patent ductus arteriosus.

Still another complication of this heart defect is the development of a blood stream infection known as subacute bacterial endocarditis, which was almost universally fatal before antibiotics, especially penicillin, came into use.

What can be done about patent ductus arteriosus? Surgery has been miraculously successful. The surgeon closes the patent ductus by tying one or two strings, or ligatures, around it and then cutting across the ductus between the two ligatures. The result is usually a heart as normal as any other, provided the operation has been done before the heart has enlarged too greatly or before the blood vessels of the lungs have narrowed. Delay until these changes develop increases the danger of the operation and makes the outcome poor.

ATRIAL SEPTAL DEFECT

Atrial septal defect is simply a hole in the wall of the septum between the right and left atria (3, diagram).

How does an atrial septal defect handicap the circulation? With each heartbeat, pure blood flows from the left atrium to the right atrium because, as previously described, the pressure in the left atrium is higher than that in the right atrium. Since pure blood is mixed with impure blood, the patient is not blue. Moreover, this condition makes the pump quite inefficient because the right ventricle must now pump this extra blood through the lungs a second time.

Furthermore, the small blood vessels in the lungs may also become narrowed and thus add to the burden of an already overworked right ventricle. Meanwhile the pressure in the right atrium has increased and soon the impure blood from the right atrium spills over into the left atrium, through the hole in the septum, finally resulting in cyanosis.

What can be done about an atrial septal defect? The hole in the septum can be closed, either by stitching the edges together or by sewing a patch of plastic material to the edges of the defect. This patch of plastic material that closes the hole is a substance foreign to the human body, but it will serve as a bridge across which living cells will grow and replace the patch. Eventually the foreign material itself will disappear.

VENTRICULAR SEPTAL DEFECT

A ventricular septal defect is a hole in the septum between the right and left ventricles (6, diagram). How does a ventricular septal defect affect the circulation? As in the atrial septal defect and patent ductus arteriosus, blood flows through the hole from the left ventricle to the right ventricle. Again both ventricles must do double duty and again the small blood vessels in the lungs may become blocked and add to the burden of the right heart.

What can be done about a ventricular septal defect? A ventricular septal defect can be closed in a manner similar to that used to correct an atrial septal defect, but in this case surgery is possible only with the aid of a heart-lung oxygenator.

ANOMALOUS PULMONARY VENOUS DRAINAGE

The pulmonary veins that carry the purified blood from the lungs (8, diagram) should normally be connected with the left atrium. Sometimes, however, some of the veins are connected with the right atrium or with one of the large veins that bring blood to the right atrium. The result is known as anomalous pulmonary venous drainage or flow.

How does this condition affect the circulation? The symptoms of anomalous pulmonary venous drainage are like those of patent ductus or the septal defects in that some blood, which has already flowed through the lungs, must be pumped through the lungs a second time. The effects on the heart are actually the same as in these conditions. To diagnose this defect correctly, special methods of investigation such as cardiac catheterization are required.

What can be done about anomalous pulmonary venous drainage? The surgeon can transplant the involved veins back into the left atrium and so restore the circulation to its normal condition.

PULMONARY ARTERIOVENOUS FISTULA

To understand pulmonary arteriovenous fistula, we must point out that, with one exception, veins convey impure blood and arteries carry pure blood. The exception is that the pulmonary artery conducts impure blood to the lungs and the pulmonary veins return the pure blood from the lungs to the left atrium.

A connection, or fistula, between a branch of the pulmonary artery and a branch of the pulmonary vein is abnormal, and its presence will cause impure blood to mix with pure blood since the pressure is higher in the pulmonary artery than in the vein.

How does a pulmonary arteriovenous fistula handicap the circulation? At first this defect does not have any appreciable effect on the circulation, but the combination of impure and pure blood does stimulate the bone marrow and an increase in the number of red blood cells results. By the time the child is five or six years old, he probably has twice as many red cells as are normally required. This condition of increased numbers of red cells is called polycythemia and accounts for the blue appearance, conspicuous in the lips and finger tips. The finger tips themselves change in shape and size, the nails become bent, and the tips of the fingers enlarge, giving the appearance of a drumstick. The toes also develop similar distortions. These changes, called "clubbing" of the fingers and toes, occur in all congenital cardiac defects whenever impure blood mixes with pure blood.

What can be done about pulmonary arteriovenous fistula? The surgical procedure for this defect consists of removing that portion of the lung in which the fistula is located. Sometimes, though rarely, several such fistulae are scattered throughout both lungs, and the condition is fatal.

NARROWING IN THE PATH OF FLOW OF BLOOD

Any narrowing in the path of flow of the blood acts as an obstruction to the free passage of blood through the area. Congenital defects involving such narrowings include coarctation of the aorta, pulmonary stenosis, and aortic stenosis.

COARCTATION OF THE AORTA

Coarctation, meaning narrowing, of the aorta is a narrowing at a point just beyond the junction of the branches of the aorta (see 1, diagram, page 25). These branches supply blood to the arms and head.

How does coarctation of the aorta handicap the circulation? In case of coarctation of the aorta, sufficient blood cannot pass through the constriction, so that the lower part of the body must get its blood supply through vessels which detour this narrowed defect. As a result of this coarctation, the left ventricle must do extra work, and the blood pressure rises in the arms and is decreased in the lower part of the body. This congenital cardiac defect can be troublesome in several ways: a) the left ventricle through overwork enlarges and eventually fails, b) the aorta may blow out or burst, c) a stroke may result because of the high blood pressure, d) a blood stream infection is not uncommon.

What can be done about coarctation of the aorta? This defect can be corrected by operation. The surgeon puts clamps above and below the constriction, dissects the narrowed portion, and sews the ends together, so that the blood can now travel freely down the aorta to the lower part of the body. Sometimes this defect is of considerable length so that a graft, either of plastic material or a piece of an aorta of another person, must be used to bridge the gap.

PULMONARY STENOSIS

The valve located where the pulmonary artery leaves the right ventricle (5, diagram) normally consists of three little cups or cusps. Sometimes their edges are so fused together that only a small hole remains through which the blood can flow to the lungs. This defect or narrowing is called pulmonary stenosis.

How does pulmonary stenosis handicap the circulation? The narrow opening results in overwork of the right ventricle and eventually in cardiac failure.

What can be done to correct pulmonary stenosis? The condition can be remarkably helped by operation, simply by slitting the valve and making a larger hole for blood to flow through to the lungs.

AORTIC STENOSIS

Aortic stenosis is a condition quite similar to pulmonary stenosis except that it affects the aortic valve, which is situated where the aorta leaves the left ventricle (4, diagram).

How does aortic stenosis handicap the circulation? Aortic stenosis results in overwork of the left ventricle and eventually results in cardiac failure. What can be done about aortic stenosis? In case of aortic stenosis, as with other similar defects, the surgeon again enlarges the opening, so that more blood can now flow through the aortic valve.

COMBINATION OF IMPERFECT SEPARATION AND ABNORMAL NARROWING

The third class of congenital heart defects includes those in which both imperfect separation of the right and left hearts and an abnormal narrowing of a blood path are involved. The classic "blue baby," whose heart malformation is known medically as the tetralogy of Fallot, is the best example of this type of defect.

TETRALOGY OF FALLOT

Fallot was the French physician who first described this condition, and tetralogy indicates the number (four) of defects involved, which are: a) pulmonary stenosis, which impedes the flow of blood to the lungs; b) a ventricular septal defect, which allows a mixing of the blood of the right and of the left ventricles; c) an enlarged aorta, which is so situated that when the right and left ventricles contract, they both pump blood up the aorta; and d) an enlargement of the right ventricle, which is the consequence of pulmonary stenosis. About 85 per cent of children who are "blue" from birth or shortly thereafter have tetralogy of Fallot.

A unique observation made of children with Fallot's tetralogy is that when they play or exercise to the point of breathlessness, they immediately assume a squatting position. This posture, strangely enough, is not seen in any other "blue" or cyanotic congenital cardiac condition, and is a positive sign in making the correct diagnosis.

How does the tetralogy of Fallot handicap the circulation? Because of the pulmonary stenosis and the free mixing of pure and impure blood in the aorta, the heart becomes quite an inefficient pump, and thus circulation of the blood is retarded.

What can be done about the tetralogy of Fallot? Some years ago, long before the heart-lung oxygenator was devised, Dr. Helen Taussig, of Baltimore, Maryland, conceived the idea that if only more blood could be steered through the lungs of children with this condition, they would be relieved of their extreme shortness of breath and the blueness which accompanies it. She consulted her surgical colleague, Dr. Alfred Blalock, who, after considerable further experimental research, performed an operation in which he joined the left subclavian artery, which is the blood vessel going to the left arm (see 7, diagram, page 25), to the pulmonary artery. In so doing, he put into practical application the idea originated by Dr. Taussig. Many children with tetralogy of Fallot were dramatically improved, but the surgeons and physicians realized that the operation was a compromise rather than a cure: although an immediate consequence of the pulmonary stenosis was relieved, all of the other defects were unaltered. In fact, an additional defect was developed.

The Blalock-Taussig operation is now obsolete but it must not be discounted. Not only did it relieve many seriously sick children but it also served as a tremendous stimulus to cardiac surgery for other congenital, and acquired, cardiac defects. The advent of the heart-lung oxygenator has made it possible to correct all of the defects combined in Fallot's tetralogy. At the successful completion of an operation for this condition today, the flow of blood to the lungs is increased, the flow from the right ventricle to the aorta is cut off, and the ventricular septal defect is closed so that there is no longer a mixture of pure and impure blood. For all practical purposes the heart is restored to normal.

CHAPTER III

Rheumatic Heart Disease

NORMAN B. ROBERG, M.D.

RHEUMATIC HEART DISEASE, the common heart disease of childhood and youth, also threatens women in their childbearing years. Men are incapacitated by this disease when their families are young and need them most. More than a million Americans are living restricted or shortened lives because of rheumatic heart disease. This ailment is present in one school child out of every hundred. Fortunately, many children and adults with rheumatic heart disease can lead normal lives, and new medical and surgical treatments are helping many others. Most encouraging and more important, in recent years we have learned that rheumatic heart disease can be prevented.

The prevention of this disease depends upon the knowledge, alertness, and interest of parents as well as physicians. Close and continuous cooperation between them is essential.

Rheumatic heart disease is an inflammation of the valves and muscle of the heart that occurs during an attack of rheumatic fever. This inflammation can lead to the creation of scar tissue, which may deform the heart valves so that they cannot function efficiently. Scar tissue in the heart muscle may reduce its strength. The words *can* and *may* are significant. The inflammation of the heart may be mild in one person and severe in another. Some persons develop more scar tissue than do others. Mild inflammation may, therefore, result in scarring. In another person, severe inflammation of the heart may heal with little or no permanent injury.

An attack of rheumatic fever does not protect the child or adult from further attacks. People do not become "immune" after one attack, as they do after an attack of measles, mumps, or chicken pox. Certain persons and families are susceptible to rheumatic fever. Not only are they not protected by an attack, but, having had one attack, they are much more likely to suffer repeatedly from rheumatic fever. Moreover, each attack of rheumatic fever further threatens or injures the heart.

THE STREPTOCOCCUS

To eliminate rheumatic heart disease, rheumatic fever must be prevented. For this the streptococcal infection which causes rheumatic fever must be detected early and eliminated promptly. The streptococcal bacteria or germs invade principally the nose and throat. They cause most of the severe sore throats, especially those associated with high fever, earache, and swollen glands in the neck. *Strepto* comes from a Greek word meaning "twisted, like a chain." *Coccus* is from another Greek word meaning "something round or oval, like a berry." Under the microscope, these bacteria or germs are seen as round organisms joined together in long, twisted chains. Thus the streptococcus is the round germ which grows in chains. The singular of the word is used generally as: "The streptococcus causes rheumatic fever." However, when many of the germs are included, the plural streptococci is used: "The throat culture showed many streptococci." The adjective, or descriptive term, is streptococcal: "The child has a streptococcal sore throat." In medical slang, streptococcal sore throat is sometimes shortened to "strep throat." Since the streptococcal infection is the cause of rheumatic fever, and penicillin kills the streptococcus, the key to the prevention of rheumatic fever is the prompt and thorough treatment of streptococcal infections with penicillin or a similar antibiotic drug.

Streptococcal infections can be suspected from the nature of the illness. The proof, however, depends upon obtaining some streptococci from the nose or throat and growing or culturing them in the laboratory. The streptococci are secured by swabbing a sterile piece of cotton over the inflamed tissues of the throat and nose. This cotton swab, which is now covered with mucus, pus, and germs, is rubbed over a culture plate that contains substances on which streptococci grow well. The culture plate is kept in an incubator at the temperature of the human body for 24 hours. If streptococci are present in the throat, they will grow on the culture plate and can be identified in the laboratory. Certainty that streptococci are present or absent cannot be established without the proof of the nose and throat culture.

A diagnosis of a streptococcal sore throat is probable if the symptoms include a rapidly developed high fever, severe pain in swallowing, and tender swollen glands below the jaw. The throat is bright red and swollen, and the back of the throat and the tonsils are flecked with pus. Usually this infection is not accompanied by a cough or runny nose. In small children the streptococcal sore throat may develop more gradually, with less fever and with a runny nose.

Viruses, which are different from bacteria such as the streptococcus, also cause sore throats. The virus infections are usually milder. The temperature is lower, pain in swallowing is mild, and the glands of the neck are not so tender and swollen. There is more coughing, the nose may run, and the entire body may ache. The virus infections are not affected by penicillin, other antibiotic drugs, or the sulfa drugs. Finally, virus infections do not cause rheumatic fever.

Streptoccal infections are passed from one person to another in the secretions of the nose and throat. Coughing throws large drops of watery mucus into the air which carry the germs with them. Sneezing spreads more streptococci than does coughing. For instance, when a person sneezes, a fine spray is forced out of the nose under high pressure and the air is heavily contaminated with germs. In the family, mucus from the nose and throat is passed from one person to another during play, kissing, and the care of the sick child. When sore throats and colds occur repeatedly within a family, a member of the family should be suspected of being a "carrier" of the streptococcus. A carrier is a person who has germs living and growing within the nose and throat without being sick and without having any signs of an infection. The nose and throat of the mother or maid or father may have become infected while taking care of a sick child. Though these persons may not become ill, they may, during kissing or playing, spread the germs to other children. One or another of these children then becomes sick. After the child has recovered from the sore throat, he may continue to have streptococci in his throat, and spread them again to other persons. Thus streptococcal infections can be passed back and forth in a family or their associates for weeks and months. When a family "has someone sick almost all the time with a sore throat or a cold," the physician often suspects that a carrier is repeatedly infecting the other members of the family. Under such circumstances, physicians often make cultures of the nose and throat of each member of the family, including those who do not show signs of infection. Antibiotic treatment is then given to everyone whose throat culture reveals streptococci.

The removal of the tonsils does not prevent streptococcal infections. Tonsils are removed, however, when they are chronically diseased. Obviously streptococci cannot any longer invade tonsils if they have been completely removed. The streptococci can, nevertheless, invade and infect the throat and the nose.

How often does a streptococcal sore throat cause rheumatic fever? In epidemics, if the streptococcal sore throat is not treated, 3 out of every 100 children and young adults develop rheumatic fever. When streptococcal infections occur in smaller numbers or are nonepidemic, the risk is less. The danger of rheumatic fever is positive every time a patient has a streptococcal sore throat. Certain persons and families have greater tendencies to develop rheumatic fever following streptococcal infections. A test or examination to determine which people are susceptible to rheumatic fever and which are not has not yet been found. This increased sensitivity to rheumatic fever is demonstrated by patients who have already had one attack: If such a patient contracts a streptococcal infection, the risk of another attack of rheumatic fever is 30 to 50 per cent. Therefore, two factors lead to rheumatic fever: the streptococcal infection and the susceptibility of the person to develop rheumatic fever. As yet, a person's tendency to develop rheumatic fever cannot be changed, but the streptococcal infection may be prevented from causing the attack. If one member of the family has had rheumatic fever or is known to have rheumatic heart disease, other members of that family may have the same tendency. If a person has had one attack of rheumatic fever, he is susceptible to recurrent attacks, and must be guarded against any chance of streptococcal infection. Such persons regularly are given small doses of penicillin or sulfonamide to keep the streptococci from invading the nose and throat. Treatment should be started immediately and not delayed until an infection is present.

The streptococcus does not directly invade the heart and joints when it causes rheumatic fever. When the streptococci germs multiply in the nose and throat, they are believed to form a product which is absorbed into the body. This substance causes the inflammation of rheumatic fever by a reaction which is similar to an allergy. Some persons, once exposed to the pollens of ragweed or grass, to egg white, or to horse serum, develop attacks of asthma, hay fever, or hives when they are again exposed to the same substance. In rheumatic fever, if the product of the streptococci continues to circulate in the body, inflammation results. If the streptococci are destroyed by penicillin before this product has been made for more than five to seven days, rheumatic fever is discouraged and will not develop. Thus, several priceless days are available in which to recognize and treat the streptococcal infection and to prevent the onset of the dread rheumatic fever.

The attack of rheumatic fever begins two or three weeks after the onset of the streptococcal infection. The person has fever and sore throat for several days, recovers from it, feels entirely well for one or two weeks, and then suddenly becomes ill with rheumatic fever. The interval between the sore throat and the onset of the rheumatic fever is the length of time necessary for the body to develop the allergic reaction to the products of the streptococcus.

SYMPTOMS OF RHEUMATIC FEVER

Rheumatic fever, called inflammatory rheumatism or acute rheumatism in the past, was named originally because of its most striking feature of painful, red, hot, and swollen joints. This acute rheumatism of youth was known to physicians three hundred years ago. Not until one hundred fifty years ago was the connection between the rheumatism and heart disease clearly recognized. This emphasis, in the name of the disease, upon the inflammation of the joints or arthritis is unfortunate for several reasons: 1) Many persons, especially young children, do not have any inflammation of the joints. 2) The joint pain may be so mild and brief that neither the child nor the family pays attention to it. 3) Even when the joints are severely inflamed, they return to normal within several weeks without any permanent joint injury. 4) Saint Vitus' dance, or chorea, occurs when rheumatic fever affects the nervous system and may not be associated with any pains or inflammation of the joints. 5) The inflammation of the heart, which can lead to permanent heart trouble, is the significant feature of rheumatic fever. In young children, the heart is most frequently involved and these young children have less involvement of the joints. Thus the name rheumatic fever refers to a harmless feature of the disease which may not be present, and the name does not suggest the importance of the inflammation of the heart. Emphasis on the inflammation of the joints may lead to the neglect of the accompanying inflammation of the heart.

Rheumatic fever is most common between the ages of five and fifteen, although it can occur at any age. The attack usually develops abruptly two or three weeks after the streptococcal infection. The sick person has a high fever, with painful, hot swelling of one or several joints. The knees, wrists, and elbows are most frequently involved. The attack may start in one or two joints, with another joint becoming inflamed every few days. As the arthritis spreads to new joints, it subsides in those which first became inflamed.

In younger children, especially those between the ages of five and ten, rheumatic fever may develop insidiously and gradually and be deceptively mild in its symptoms. The fever may be low, and the child will be tired, anemic, and fail to gain weight. The nose may bleed repeatedly without apparent reason. Sometimes dull red blotches develop in the skin which tend to form circles. These circular areas spread outwards, leaving a clear area of skin in the center. Painless, hard lumps may develop over the bony parts of the joints, the spine, and the back of the head. Instead of having red, swollen, and painful joints, these younger children may have vague aching of the arms and legs. This vague aching raises the difficult question of whether or not these are the pains of rheumatic fever or the so-called growing pains which occur in healthy children. If a vigorous child plays hard all afternoon and then awakens at night with leg pains, these may be "growing pains." If a child is listless and refuses to play because of leg pains, rheumatic fever should be considered seriously. Aching and pain of the limbs requires careful medical examination.

Saint Vitus' dance may be the only sign of rheumatic fever, and will be followed by heart disease just as often as when the joints are inflamed. When Saint Vitus' dance is severe, the afflicted person twists, jerks, and throws the head, arms, and legs in uncontrolled and unpredictable ways. The wild motions and jerkings of the limbs, and the strange positions of the body, explain the name chorea from the Greek word meaning "dance." The common name of Saint Vitus' dance was applied to the disease in the Middle Ages because Saint Vitus was the patron saint of those who had epilepsy and nervous disorders.

Saint Vitus' dance is as much part of rheumatic fever as the inflammation of the joints. It follows streptococcal infections, and can return after new streptococcal infections. With each attack, the heart is exposed to further injury. The first signs of Saint Vitus' dance are clumsiness and emotional disturbances. The child may knock over glasses, spill food, and drop things. When chorea is more severe the child cannot control muscles of the face, the tongue, the arms, or the legs. The emotional instability often is interpreted as a behavior problem, and the parents are unhappy when they learn that they have been punishing a sick child. Most attacks of chorea last six to eight weeks, but some last six months. The development of clumsiness, jerks, and twistings of the face, irritability, and emotional instability indicates the need for careful medical evaluation. An attack of chorea, or Saint Vitus' dance, requires careful treatment and prolonged observation as does every attack of rheumatic fever, including the preventive use of the antibiotic drugs.

The severity of the symptoms and signs of rheumatic fever, whether the rheumatic form with joint pains or the nervous form with Saint Vitus' dance, does not indicate the degree of injury to the heart. Serious inflammation of the heart may accompany several months of "tiredness and pains from fallen arches." An illness characterized by piercing arthritis moving from one joint to another, or by severe Saint Vitus' dance, may be followed by complete recovery without evidence of heart disease. Although the inflamed joints, or the Saint Vitus' dance, demand immediate attention, management of the inflammation of the heart valves and heart muscle is more important though not so obvious.

The attack of rheumatic fever is not completely over when the fever, joint pains, or chorea have disappeared. In fires, the disappearance of high flames and clouds of smoke does not indicate that the fire is completely out. The fire may continue to smolder. The damage done by the smoldering embers may be far more significant than that which occurs when the flames and smoke are at their height. The fever, inflamed joints, and Saint Vitus' dance usually subside within four to eight weeks, and the child feels and looks much better. The smoldering activity of the rheumatic fever, deep within the body and within the heart, usually continues for another two to four months. Only meticulous examinations by the physician, with laboratory tests, can determine when the rheumatic fever has become inactive.

TREATMENT OF RHEUMATIC FEVER

The treatment of acute rheumatic fever is based upon rest. Once an attack of rheumatic fever has begun and the tissues have become inflamed, a particular medicine or treatment is not known as yet which will eliminate this inflammation or definitely shorten the time that it exists. When a person suffers a severe burn of the skin, a bruise, or a deep cut, he must wait until nature heals the injured and inflamed tissues. The treatments do not "heal" or "cure" these injuries, but they do aid natural healing. Placing a broken arm in a cast does not heal the broken bone. Keeping the broken bone at rest permits healing to take place rapidly. Infectious diseases such as measles, mumps, and chicken pox also must run their natural courses. Keeping the sick person at rest and using certain treatment to make him more comfortable and to prevent complications is the most that the physician can do. The same principle applies to rheumatic fever. The attack of rheumatic fever usually will heal and pass within one to four months. To keep the heart at rest, the sick child must be kept quiet. How long any patient must be kept absolutely in bed, and when some activity can be allowed, are determined by the physician's periodic examinations. Some patients must be kept in bed for several months, while others are allowed to sit up and go to the toilet within a few weeks.

Some medicines are definitely valuable in reducing the intensity of the fever, sickness, and joint inflammation; others will lessen the disturbances of Saint Vitus' dance. The medicine most widely used, and whose value is proven, is aspirin. The benefit of aspirin is not merely in the reduction of fever and pain. Aspirin, given in large amounts—from 6 to 30 tablets a day, depending upon the patient's age and condition—often eliminates the fever and arthritis within one or two days. Drugs of any kind, even aspirin, are given only under the physician's supervision. Cortisone and ACTH act like a "super" aspirin, and the patient improves dramatically. When patients receive such powerful drugs as cortisone and ACTH, they must be observed closely and ordinarily should be in a hospital.

At present definite evidence that aspirin, or cortisone and ACTH, shorten the attack of rheumatic fever or lessen the inflammation and scarring of the heart valves is not available. These medicines, especially cortisone and ACTH, will reduce abruptly the fever and the inflammation of the joints. The patient feels better and some of the laboratory tests become more normal. If the medicines are stopped, the fever, joint pains, and abnormal laboratory tests reappear. Treatment with these or with similar drugs is worthwhile and helpful, but it must be remembered that these medicines are not curative. Rather, their effect is suppressive. They suppress the inflammation but do not eliminate it. The inflammation of rheumatic fever continues to smolder quietly while the patient is under this treatment. The physician understands this and the patient and family too should comprehend, so that the necessary rest and precautions are not neglected because the patient looks and feels better and does not have pain.

A course of penicillin therapy is given when the diagnosis of rheumatic fever is made. The penicillin eliminates any streptococci which are present in the nose and throat and prevents more of the products of the streptococcus from being absorbed into the body. Some evidence indicates that the elimination of the streptococci after the attack has begun may cause the attack of rheumatic fever to be milder. The benefits of cortisone, ACTH, and penicillin, when given during the first week or two of the attack, are being investigated. At present, from the practical aspect of the patient's management, these drugs are unquestioningly considered valuable to some patients. Nevertheless, they do not "cure" the rheumatic fever and do not diminish the need for rest and close observation.

The rheumatic fever patient must not be allowed to have additional streptococcal infections. With each such new infection, he will have a 50 per cent chance of another attack of rheumatic fever. If the heart escapes damage with the first attack, it may be injured during the second. If the heart has been injured in the first attack of rheumatic fever, further inflammation and scarring will be added to the damage already present. New infections by streptococci, and repeated attacks of rheumatic fever, can be prevented by penicillin or the sulfonamides.

When one of these drugs is used to destroy the streptococci which are present and causing infection, the procedure is called penicillin therapy, or therapeutic penicillin. The terms therapy and therapeutic mean treatment. When penicillin is used to prevent streptococci from entering and infecting the throat, this use is called penicillin prophylaxis, or prophylactic penicillin. The words prophylaxis and prophylactic mean "to guard against." The difference between these two uses of penicillin is important. Penicillin therapy is prescribed when a patient has a streptococcal infection, such as a streptococcal sore throat. It is also prescribed to rid the patient of any streptococci which are present in the nose and throat after the infection has passed. Penicillin prophylaxis is prescribed when it is important to prevent streptococci from invading the nose and the throat. The therapeutic dose is much larger than the prophylactic dose. The patient who has had an attack of rheumatic fever should receive prophylactic penicillin so that streptococci cannot invade the throat and nose and manufacture the products that will cause another attack of rheumatic fever. Thus prophylactic penicillin is given to a patient who does not have a streptococcal infection, does not have any streptococci in the nose or throat, but as a "rheumatic fever patient" cannot risk getting another streptococcal infection.

A serious complication of rheumatic heart disease is bacterial endocarditis. This ailment is a direct invasion of the injured heart valves by bacteria circulating in the blood stream. During childbirth, the extraction of teeth, or the removal of diseased tonsils, bacteria or germs get into the blood stream. Normal persons promptly destroy these germs. But in rheumatic fever patients, these germs may gain a foothold on the injured heart valves. To prevent this complication, such patients are given large amounts of penicillin or other antibiotic drugs before and after the removal of either teeth or tonsils. Such a patient who is pregnant is given the drug before she goes into labor. These large additional doses are given to persons who are already receiving regular prophylactic penicillin.

When anyone develops acute rheumatic fever, therapeutic penicillin is given to destroy the streptococci that remain in the nose or throat. After these streptococci are eliminated, prophylactic penicillin is started so that new streptococci cannot gain a foothold and begin a new attack. Prophylactic penicillin should be initiated and maintained during the acute onset of rheumatic fever, and should be continued during the convalescence and after the patient has recovered. Prophylactic penicillin is started promptly so that members of the family or visitors who may have a streptococcal infection, or who may be carriers of the germs, do not reinfect the patient. After the attack is over and the patient resumes a normal life, the prophylactic penicillin protects him from contracting a streptococcal infection from people who are sneezing and coughing in school, in offices, in public places, in buses and street cars.

When or where the rheumatic fever patient may be exposed to someone who is spreading streptococci cannot be known or anticipated. True streptococcal infections are less frequent in the summer and in the southern part of the United States. Although less chance of contracting an infection prevails in certain seasons and in some places, the rheumatic fever patient is never completely safe from another streptococcal infection, regardless of season or place. No child or adult can be protected from streptococcal infection by the impractical advice, "stay away from crowds." Penicillin prophylaxis will protect them, however, and will permit them to lead normal lives without fear of new infections.

Penicillin prophylaxis can be maintained either by injection of a particular kind of penicillin once a month or by taking tablets twice each day. The monthly injection of the long-lasting type of penicillin, although it may require a visit to the physician and an injection in the buttock, offers many advantages:

1) The injection is more dependable and prevents 99 per cent of streptococcal infections; penicillin taken by mouth protects against only 95 per cent of infections. The difference does not seem great, but it can be all-important to the person who has recurrent rheumatic fever.

2) The absorption of penicillin from the stomach is not complete, and the amount absorbed of any dose varies from person to person; therefore large amounts must be given by mouth to make sure that enough will be absorbed. The cost of the penicillin tablets for a month is about five times the cost of the penicillin to be injected. When the physician's fee for giving the injection is included, the injection is still no more expensive than the tablets.

3) The injection insures maximal protection for an entire month. The patient and his family are relieved of the responsibility of making sure that the tablets are taken twice a day, every day, every month.

4) The patient, especially if young, is impressed with the importance of preventing any recurrent streptococcal infection by the regular visit to his doctor. Responsibility for the prophylaxis is preferably vested in the physician, so that the child cannot accuse his family of "always nagging—never letting me alone" in this connection.

5) The periodic examination of the heart and the necessary laboratory tests can be performed by the physician at the same time that the injections are given.

6) If the first attack of rheumatic fever has resulted in some injury to the heart valves or the heart muscle, the monthly visits give the patient an opportunity to discuss problems with the physician and give him the occasion to instruct the patient in further details of understanding his condition and caring for himself.

7) If the patient is a child or adolescent, a great psychological ad-

vantage is developed in going to the doctor's office once a month; he goes "for my injection" and not "because I have a bad heart."

To sum up, the monthly injections of penicillin serve two major purposes: The injection prevents further streptococcal infections and thereby prevents recurrent attacks of rheumatic fever and progressive damage to the heart. The monthly visits to the physician, which start in the convalescent period, educate the patient to the recognition and acceptance of being "a rheumatic fever patient." For anyone who has had an attack of rheumatic fever must accept the fact that he is a "rheumatic fever patient" for the rest of his life.

The education of the rheumatic fever patient has three principal features: 1) the necessity of avoiding further attacks of rheumatic fever; 2) the importance of avoiding needless invalidism and limitations of activity; 3) the careful supervision of activity and treatment of rheumatic heart disease that results from rheumatic fever.

Rheumatic fever is most likely to recur within the first five years following the first attack. It is most recurrent during youth, and the attacks are less frequent after the age of thirty. The rheumatic fever patient must, therefore, receive prophylactic penicillin for the first five years following the attack, and should continue to receive prophylactic penicillin until the age of thirty, even if the evidence of rheumatic heart disease seems to have disappeared. If rheumatic heart disease has developed, it may be best for the patient to continue to receive penicillin the rest of his life.

The avoidance of unnecessary invalidism and the comprehension of the limitations that must be respected in order to lead as normal a life as the condition of the heart will allow are important. Heart murmurs are the prime evidence that rheumatic heart disease has developed during the attack of rheumatic fever. However, the heart murmur heard during the attack of rheumatic fever does not always signify with certainty that the person has rheumatic heart disease. Some heart murmurs do not imply disease, and such harmless murmurs can be heard in 30 to 50 per cent of normal children and adolescents. Thus the murmur heard during an attack of rheumatic fever may be a normal murmur—may have always been present, and may be unrelated to the attack of rheumatic fever. Some murmurs during the acute stage of rheumatic fever are simply the result of fever and anemia and disappear when these symptoms disappear. In certain instances the heart valves may be temporarily stretched and swollen, and they will return to normal within a few weeks or months. The future of the heart cannot be predicted from the murmur heard during the acute phase of rheumatic fever.

About 60 per cent of rheumatic fever patients will develop a murmur which indicates definite rheumatic heart disease. The stream of blood rushing through a valve which has become scarred causes the murmur. The presence of a murmur does not indicate that rheumatic fever is still active and that the patient must remain quiet. For example, when the appendix has been removed in case of acute appendicitis, a scar remains on the abdomen. This scar does not imply that the patient still has acute appendicitis. A heart murmur resulting from rheumatic heart disease signifies that a scar has remained after the acute attack, but it does not imply that the heart and its valves are still inflamed. The presence of a murmur indicating rheumatic heart disease does not, in itself, mean invalidism and a life of limited activity.

The problems relating to the interpretation of heart murmurs indicate the significance of the periodic examinations following acute rheumatic fever.

These questions are among those most usually asked of doctors about rheumatic heart disease:

If a murmur develops during the acute attack, does it disappear promptly? If the murmur persists, is it one of the normal murmurs, or is it one of the murmurs that indicates rheumatic heart disease? If it is definitely a murmur of rheumatic heart disease, does it imply mild, moderate, or severe injury to the heart valve? Which valve is involved, and is more than one valve injured? Has the strength of the heart muscle been impaired? How much activity may the patient undertake without placing a strain upon the heart? Shall this child be allowed to compete in certain athletics? Is it safe for that young woman to become pregnant?

Exactly the same condition does not pertain in any two patients with rheumatic heart disease. Some patients live a long and active life, while others may develop progressive narrowing of a heart valve which obstructs blood flow and, after many years, will demand an operation to open the valve. Still other types of valve disease require different treatment. The degree of heart disease, its rate of progress, and the relationship to the patient's daily life cannot be predicted at the time of the attack of rheumatic fever. During the months and years that follow the attack, the physician must evaluate regularly the progress of the disease and advise the patient according to the results of these examinations.

The majority of patients with rheumatic heart disease can lead normal lives. With modern knowledge and treatment, most women with rheumatic heart disease can have safely the number of children that they wish. Although most patients with rheumatic heart disease should avoid strenuous sports, exercise is good for these particular patients; exercise, but not strain and fatigue, is good for the body and for the heart. Most of the patients can bowl, golf, garden, dance, walk, swim, and row. By knowledge of themselves, and with the advice of their physicians, they can lead full and active lives.

Modern treatment and methods of diagnosis have greatly changed the outlook for patients with rheumatic heart disease. The details of therapy, and the needs of each patient, are decided individually, according to the particular conditions and needs of that person. The great advance in medicine has been the solving of the relationship of streptococcal infections to rheumatic fever, and the ability to prevent rheumatic fever by treatment with penicillin. Someday a method may be found by which patients can be vaccinated against streptococcal infections, and then even penicillin management and prophylaxis would become unnecessary. For the time being, the advance against rheumatic fever and rheumatic heart disease has been successful. They are definitely preventable. The identification and prompt treatment of streptococcal infections and the prevention of further similar infections are the keys to the conquest of rheumatic heart disease. Inevitably, certain mild streptococcal infections and some mild cases of rheumatic fever will not be detected, and rheumatic heart disease will occur. But the knowledge and the means of preventing most rheumatic heart disease are already available. The close cooperation between the family and the physician can prevent rheumatic fever, can lessen its damage to the heart if it does occur, and can prevent future attacks. Prevention is the goal, and it can be attained.

Chapter IV

Living Along Well with Coronary Artery Disease

George R. Herrmann, M.D.

Great numbers of men in their most productive years continue to be active without symptoms and are totally unaware of the presence of significant and potentially dangerous coronary artery disease. Many others who have suffered attacks of angina pectoris or coronary thrombosis are living comfortable, happy lives, having slightly modified their ways of life. The modifications depend on the person's psychic and physical make-up, his habits, occupation, and economic status. The intelligent patients who have learned every known fact about coronary artery disease and thrombosis, and have been particularly cooperative, have been easily and successfully managed and have enjoyed longevity.

CURRENT CONCEPTS OF ATHEROSCLEROSIS

The causes of atherosclerosis, and for its strategic localization in the coronary arteries, are unknown. Atherosclerosis is not the unavoidable accompaniment of natural aging—it is definitely premature aging. Many factors are recognized that contribute to the production and growth of subintimal arterial lesions, that is, lesions under the inner lining of the blood vessels. Members of a family in which one person is affected should be alerted to their hereditary predisposition to atherosclerosis. Such awareness justifies the practice of avoiding or curbing recognized causative or aggravating factors and the atherogenic precipitating habits.

Habits that are predisposing, perpetuating, and precipitating are excessive drive, aggressiveness, overambition, tension, exposure to emotional stresses and strains, and dietary indiscretions such as indulgence in rich, high-caloric animal and dairy fats. Hypercholesterolemia, or high blood-cholesterol levels, should be carefully watched, and the level lowered if found to be excessive. Obesity, or overweight, although not definitely incriminated in atheromatosis should be reduced. Sedentary indolence does not, in itself, seem to be conducive to atherosclerosis, and some physical activity, such as walking or bicycling, is desirable. Exercise after eating a rich meal tends to reduce the blood fat levels. The nicotine of tobacco, in smoking or chewing, is a more powerful vasoconstrictor and therefore the use of tobacco should be sharply curtailed.

High blood fat levels of cholesterol, phospholipids, large chylomicrons, beta lipoproteins, triglycerides, and the lighter, more slowly centrifuged-down fatty molecules have been found to be associated with atheromatous disease of the coronary arteries in man. It is not yet established which lipid fraction is most atherogenic to start or add to a fatty plaque in a coronary artery wall. Several theoretical reasons have been offered for the localization and growth of the fatty plaques in the subintima, just under the lining of the arteries, especially at strategic points of the coronaries and large branches of the aorta.

The great sex factor or the greater frequency of premature aging in men as contrasted to women up to the age of the menopause has been variously explained. The thinner intima of the coronary arteries in women was considered to prevent the passage of lipids while the thicker intima of men was thought to be a less efficient barrier. However, the estrogen level changes at menopause with the accompanying rise of the more atherogenic beta lipoproteins is considered to be a cause for the unusually high incidence of atherosclerosis in men and the increased incidence in women after menopause.

Blood pressure elevations are more common in men and seemingly contribute to coronary artery disease. The greater turbulence and pressures on the intima at angulations of arteries may mechanically drive the lipids through the intima, and initiate and contribute to fatty plaque formation and growth. However, other serum constituents as albumin, fibrin, and fibrinolysins, as well as lipids may be mechanically driven into and through the lining of the arteries at the heavily buffeted points. According to other investigators, there are active metabolic processes with affinities for lipids going on in the arterial wall, and lipids are synthesized in the arterial wall and pass back and forth across the intimal membrane.

A few investigators have felt that more or less insoluble cholesterol crystals and grumous lipids in the subintimal tissue have resulted from local cellular necrosis and/or degeneration of local intramural hemorrhage and blood clot formation. The sudden swelling of an atheromatous plaque to the point of occluding a coronary artery has been established by pathologists as a common cause for sudden death, as has erosion of the intima and a resulting thrombosis of a large branch of a coronary artery. Local tissue fibrinolysins have been demonstrated in atheromatous plaques. Sudden rises in blood pressure as a result of extreme exertion or physical strain or sustained effort may produce intramural hemorrhage and sudden swelling of the atheromatous plaque. A split in the intima may start a thrombosis and thus contribute to arterial occlusion and myocardial infarction.

High blood fat levels, or hyperlipemia, have been shown to facilitate intra-arterial clotting by inhibiting fibrinolysins and to be accompanied by sludging and coagulation of the blood, especially if the circulation is slowed. Dietary indiscretions, particularly a high intake of animal fat and dairy products (especially butter and cream) that contain a high percentage of saturated fats, will cause and maintain high blood lipid levels and encourage thrombosis. Impaired liver function may mobilize lipid from fat deposits to produce hypercholesterolemia. Lowered thyroid function and other endocrinopathies may give rise to fat mobilizing factors as that from the posterior pituitary gland. Several investigators have gotten evidence that emotional stress and strain may produce significal elevations in blood lipid levels depending some upon the individual's inborn neuroendocrine metabolic response to the stress.

Any occupation may be the source of emotional stress to the susceptible aggressive, ambitious person who strives for advancement in this competitive life and who with attainment of his goal has assumed added responsibility. The compulsive, unrestrained urge calls forth superhuman efforts, suppression of personal discomforts, disregard of health maxims, and neglect of induced fatigue. Fatigue and excitation drives the victim on to nervous exhaustion. These activities all contribute, as do domestic squabbles with emotional strain and outbursts of anger, to increased epinephrine or adrenal secretion and blood pressure elevation. Epinephrine or adrenalin may accelerate cholesterol and phospholipid depositions in the intima, the lining of the blood vessels. Catecholamine phospholipids have been shown to have an affinity for arterial tissues and to produce injury to the intima and vasoconstriction.

Emotional stresses affect the higher nervous tissue and by brain and hormonal mechanisms may cause, in addition to the arterial intimal injury, elevation of the blood fats, decreased fluidity, and increased coagulability of the blood. These must be avoided to insure a comfortable way of life such as is conducive to longevity.

The attending physician and the patient who is found to be a candidate for, or who has sustained, a coronary thrombosis should have some idea of the procedures that are thought to prevent coronary artery disease, atheromatosis, and thrombosis. The clearer the concept that the patient has of the disease, the more intelligently and willingly will he cooperate in the readjustments of his life that may seem necessary to halt or slow down progression of the disease processes and prevent the complications.

Each patient presents some individual problems that must be solved for him by his physician. However, there are many contributing factors to atheromatosis that are common to most patients with coronary artery disease, so that some generally applicable health rules or preventive measures may be advantageous to most patients. Most patients need some advice as to how to live more sanely or reasonably and how to conduct their affairs effectively with care and the hope and assurance of rewards of many years of comfort. Any sense of fear, inadequacy, and insecurity must be allayed and personal contentment assured.

The way of life that a given person may follow depends upon the extent of damage that his heart muscle has sustained as a result of the coronary thrombosis. How much heart muscle has been destroyed, how well has the infarct healed and the dead heart muscle been absorbed and replaced by scar tissue? How extensive and how adequate a collateral circulation has developed? What, if any, complications have developed in the scarring, and how much good functioning heart muscle remains? Gradually the patient should be made to understand just what his condition is, but it is rarely necessary to be blunt or brutal. The answer to these questions are apparent to the patient's physician and are reflected in the patient's exercise tolerance.

A patient may, of course, survive several attacks of coronary thrombosis, but each attack decreases his heart muscle mass and his reserve and his life span. Therefore every effort should be made to prevent recurrences and complications.

The very important period of convalescence from an acute attack of coronary thrombosis is most contributory to longevity. Most careful management is required to insure recovery with the minimum of complications. Good care during the acute attack may add years of comfort. Intelligent rest in bed should be required for at least four weeks. Recurrent coronary pain may be relieved by narcotics at first. Anxiety, apprehension, fear, nervous tension, and restlessness may be allayed by sedatives and reassurance. Cardiac mechanism disorders and metabolic diseases such as myxedema, diabetes mellitus, and hypercholesterolemia should be gotten under control as soon as possible. Blood sludging and increased coagulability if present should be decreased with heparin and anticoagulants prescribed by the doctor. The patient's blood pressure should be maintained above 100 and below 140 mm. Hg.

The patient is instructed to lie flat in bed, with elevation of his head to the point of comfortable breathing. His trunk should be turned by the nurse and passive exercises of his legs and arms should be carried out by an attendant at least four times a day for ten to twenty minutes each time if the patient tolerates it well. In the third and fourth week of uneventful convalescence, the patient should be calmly advised about his condition, his re-education begun, and his program for succeeding weeks, months, and years outlined. Very gradually, physical activity is increased, as sitting slightly in bed and for longer periods day by day with the moving of extremities. Dropping the legs over the side of the bed may be started in the fifth week. Most patients should be allowed to sit on the side of the bed and begin gradually and slowly to assume the upright position for longer periods and take some steps in the sixth week and the rehabilitation begins in the seventh week. If essential hypertension returns, the physician should reduce the blood pressure to normal and maintain it so with anti-hypertensive drugs.

Most of these patients must be taught how to live a little more by the wayside as they travel on through life. The idea that their watchword must henceforth be moderation in all things must be fixed in their minds.

THE RETURN TO THE JOB

The question as to whether and when the patient is allowed to return to his job depends on many factors that vary from patient to patient. The answer can come only after consideration of all available data and information in each individual case.

Every patient should have something to occupy his mind, and most patients need to return to a financially remunerative occupation to make ends meet and to have peace of mind. The period of convalescence and rehabilitation depends upon the severity of the attack, the extent of the loss of heart muscle and the severity of complications and shock, cardiac mechanism disorders and the ease of control of paroxysms, heart block, atrial fibrillation, congestive heart failure, hypotension or persistent hypertension, and the patient's psychic reaction to his situation.

Most patients must be taught how to worry successfully, as David Seabury advocated in his book of that title. He must learn to delegate responsibility and the necessary authority and gracefully administer all matters without effort or emotion. If tenseness persists he must practice "progressive relaxation" as outlined by Edmund Jacobson in his book, *You Must Relax*. The return to work is dependent upon the patient's state of recovery, attitude or mental adjustment, exercise tolerance, and financial resources. Chronic physical invalidism or retirement may be suggested if the patient and/or his family can afford it and if he can be taught to enjoy it, or if symptoms totally disable and plague him upon every mental and physical effort.

After four to six months, partial resumption of his occupation on a half-time basis for six months may be permitted to many patients, particularly if his work is sedentary and not exciting and can be carried out without bringing on pain or breathlessness. The patient's idea that everything, including life itself, depends upon his holding the job must be dispelled and the patient's viewpoint reoriented. Heavy work or occupations that require quick or prolonged physical or mental effort under pressure or deadlines of time cannot be resumed, and vocational training in a less demanding activity should be advised. At any job during the first year, each two hours of physical or mental effort should be complemented by a rest period; after four hours, a siesta, a midday reclining on a cot, couch, or bed for at least one hour, should be prescribed.

Unfavorable reactions to the patient's gradual return to a modified activity with curtailed hours, such as rising blood pressure levels, recurrent attacks of pain or breathlessness or palpitation, nervous tension states, exhaustion or jitteriness, call for another rest period of six months and then later another trial of gradual resumption of activities.

TREATMENT

General measures to modify the fairly well established predisposing, perpetuating, and precipitating factors of the disease should be undertaken during the convalescence and rehabilitation and carried on throughout life thereafter.

In addition to the psychologic approaches, the patient, if he has a tendency to blood clot formation, is maintained on anticoagulants over a period of years and sometimes indefinitely if he tolerates the drugs. Coronary vasodilators, such as slowly released nitroglycerin and tetranitrates (erythrol) in sublingual preparations, are widely used. Niacin and aminophyllin likewise are used to improve coronary blood flow and prevent or relieve recurrent pain.

DIET

If the person is obese, weight should be gradually reduced at the rate of a pound a week to the ideal for his height. In addition to the reduction in total caloric intake, the contributory role of hyperlipemia is so well established that the intake of calories from fats should be reduced to not more than 30 per cent of the total calories of the diet, and of this 30 per cent, two-thirds should be of unsaturated fatty acids, nonhydrogenated oil of corn, soya, sesame, cottonseed, peanuts, and olives and not more than one-third of saturated animal, dairy, poultry, or hydrogenated vegetable fats. Palatable and satisfactory meals may be prepared, observing these rules and by following the suggestions of Ancel and Margaret Keys in their book, *Eat Well and Stay Well*. These moderate dietary restrictions must be practiced year in and year out.

Persistently high blood-serum lipid levels warrant the administration of thyroid extract in those with hypometabolism, and estrogen, a female sex hormone, in the patients after the menopause, and possibly in men with very high beta lipoprotein ratios who respond to non-feminizing hormones satisfactorily without experiencing distressing side effects.

Nicotinic acid in high dosage, 3 to 9 grams per day, has been shown to reduce blood lipid levels presumably by oxidation, but in spite of slowly released niacin the flushing and itching may be unbearable. Swiss, French, and Mexican investigators have used P.E.A.A. (phenyl ethyl acetoamide) to depress cholesterol synthesis in the liver with some success. In spite of all these efforts, the dietary restriction of the excessive intake of saturated fats and the substitution of unsaturated fatty acids to the extent of 20 per cent of the allowable total 30 per cent of the fat calories seems to be the most promising long-term method of attacking the problem.

ACCESSORY PRACTICES CONDUCIVE TO LONGEVITY

Eating should be done in a calm, quiet, cheerful atmosphere in pleasant surroundings, when the patient is relaxed and rested. The noon meal should be the main meal of the day and supper be just a light, easily digested snack. Heavy eating late at night and banquets are to be avoided. Iced or frosted, highly carbonated cold drinks should be sipped only in small swallows and held in the mouth until warm before swallowing. Alcoholic beverages in moderation before dinner or after meals and at bedtime may often be of medicinal value. Salt should be sharply restricted especially in those patients with hypertension or a tendency to edema. Coffee and tea should be restricted and decaffeinated drinks substituted.

Political or business conference with the meals are an abomination and should be prohibited. After-dinner speaking invitations should be rejected. The use of tobacco in any form should be interdicted immediately, especially if the patient is hypersensitive, and at least sharply reduced and restricted unless withdrawal creates a psychic storm. Arguments and attempts at convincing others, even friends, or of outwitting a competitor, or wearing opposition down causes stress and blood pressure rise and should be avoided. Great tenacity of purpose causes emotional strain and should be tempered down. Work and play should be so planned or scheduled that everything may be accomplished in the time allotted without attempting to meet sharp "deadlines" for production. Relaxed slow motion like that of "Lazy Bones" or Stepin Fetchit should be emulated.

Exercise such as walking or bicycling on level ground for several blocks to a mile should be carried out daily, but sudden starts, dashing or running, or uphill grinds should be avoided. Stairs, if they must be climbed, should be mounted one half-step at a time. Driving an automobile in heavy traffic and parallel parking are usually strenuous as are intensely competitive games as golf, tennis, and baseball. Most sports are too exciting even when viewed on television and may precipitate coronary trouble.

Most patients can tolerate elevations to 5,000 feet, if activities are minimal. Higher altitudes should be approached gradually and supplementary oxygen by mask taken if dyspnea is experienced. Flying in planes that are usually pressurized at 5,000 feet is perfectly safe as oxygen and masks are available in most modern aircraft and may be requested and used if desired.

Still pole fishing, sit-down bait casting or trolling, and hunting from a blind or in level meadows are good recreational activities if all the strenuous physical efforts of arranging for the expedition are entrusted to others.

Regular breaks should be arranged in the daily program. Vacations and recreations should be taken as necessary healthful interludes regularly, frequently, in a leisurely way with complete relaxation and not regimented or filled with more things to do than can be done and not considered a waste of time or regarded as unnecessary or too costly. All work and troubles are to be left in the office or at the plant when the day's work is done and not carried home or on pleasure trips or returned to on week ends.

The patient must curb his overambition and change his outlook upon life. He needs to cultivate his sense of humor, to walk away from and avoid all situations fraught with dangerous turmoil, noise, confusion, strain, excitement, and agitation. Instead, he should cultivate relaxation, calmness, quiet, composure, order, and rhythm in all activities. He must learn to economize on physical and mental effort, practice restraint, and create in himself an imperturbable state of mind.

The patient should build in and about himself an environment of tranquillity and an air of serenity at his work and in his home so that he may fully relax in body and enjoy an equanimity of mind and soul.

He should make his physician his advisor and counselor, consult him regularly, and abide by his advice.

Chapter V

The Heart Muscle

Morris W. Stroud III, M.D.

The heart is composed almost entirely of muscle. The rate and force of pumping are controlled by specialized muscular tissue. The right side of the heart pumps blood through the lungs where carbon dioxide is eliminated and oxygen absorbed. The left side of the heart pumps blood to all the tissues of the body. If the heart stops for more than three to five minutes, irreversible changes take place in the brain and later in other organs. Therefore, the heart muscles never cease pumping twenty-four hours a day. The heart muscle is a tough, durable material which is more resistant to lack of oxygen, diseases, and toxic agents than any other vital organ in the body. Since man first began studying the human body scientifically, the heart and particularly heart muscle have been studied intensely, more perhaps than any other part of the body in regard to structure, response to drugs, biochemistry, metabolism, and reaction to stress and disease.

MUSCLE FIBERS

The composition of the individual fibers of the heart muscle is different from that of skeletal and smooth muscle. Until recently it was thought that the individual fibers of the cardiac muscle blended into each other. Actually, each fiber is a discrete unit. These units are small; the normal diameter ranging from 12.5 to 14.0 micrometers or 1/2000 inch. In the atria, or auricles, the muscular walls are rather thin. In the ventricles, the walls are quite thick, being thickest in the walls of the left ventricle, particularly at its base. There are four fairly discrete muscle groups in the ventricles. Each muscle has a specific function. The two superficial muscles fix the fulcrums of the heart so that the wall between the two ventricles and the thin-walled apexes do not bulge during the expulsion of blood from the ventricles. They also set the heart valves and thus prevent backward leakage of blood. The deep sinospiral muscle is responsible for emptying the right ventricle, and it also plays a significant part in the early emptying of the left ventricle. The deep bulbospiral muscle, which forms the base of the left ventricle, provides the principal expulsive force of the left ventricle. Its action in wringing out the last portion of blood left in the ventricle is similar to the clenching of the fist. This muscle is vitally important. Survival is possible even if both superficial muscles and/or the deep sinospiral are injured, but animals studied have never survived when the deep bulbospiral muscle was severely damaged.

HOW THE HEART BEATS

The heart provides its own ignition. The sparkplug is the pacemaker, also known as the sinoauricular node, sinoatrial node, or more briefly, the SA node. This nerve center is a tiny island of specialized neuro-muscular tissue located in the right atrium near the vena cava. The atrioventricular node, abbreviated as the AV node, is located in the interatrial septum near the junction of the atria and the ventricles. It forms the head of a specialized neuromuscular tissue, known as the Purkinje network, which passes through the fibrous ring that separates the atria and ventricles. The AV node splits into two discrete bundles as it progresses down the ventricular septum and then, by branching extensively, sweeps around the ventricles and back towards the base of the heart where the deep bulbospiral muscle is located. When the SA node fires, it sets off an electrical impulse that travels so rapidly through the atria to the AV node that the two atria simultaneously eject blood into the ventricles. There is a pause in the forward wave of electrical excitation at the AV node, which enables the atrioven-tricular valves to close before the ventricles contract. The total time between the firing of the SA node and the start of the electrical wave in the AV node is from 0.12 to 0.22 seconds. From the AV node, the current travels rapidly down the Purkinje network through the bundle of His, the right and left bundles in the interventricular septum, and then through the branching fibers to the four ventricular muscles. The last area to be excited is the base of the left ventricle.

Any part of the heart muscle will contract and relax at a regular rate if isolated from other sources of stimulation. Tissue cultures of heart muscle maintain this characteristic feature indefinitely. The intrinsic rate is fastest in the SA node and progressively slower in atrial muscle, AV node, and the ventricles. The SA-node firing rate is controlled by the relative influence of the two autonomic nerves that conduct impulses from the brain to the heart. Impulses from the vagus nerve slow the heart rate by depressing rhythmicity of the SA node and by slowing the conduction rate through the AV node. The vagus nerve has little if any action upon the force of contraction. The sympathetic nerve fibers, or accelerator nerves, increase the rate of the SA node, speed the conduction through the AV node, and increase the force and rate of contraction of the muscle fibers. The velocity of contraction is so accelerated that the heart actually spends more time per minute in diastole, or the resting state, than before the sympathetic stimulation. The increased amount of time spent in diastole is of great importance since the heart receives most of its blood from the coronary arteries when it is not contracting. The contracting muscles of the ventricles squeeze the coronary arteries and, furthermore, may cause backward flow in the muscle areas closest to the ventricular chambers. The heart is continually being stimulated both by the vagus and sympathetic nerve fibers, and the rate and force of contraction of the heart depends upon the relative intensity of the two nerves. The nerves receive impulses from the brain centers, which are continually receiving messages from the vast sensory system spread throughout the body. In addition, strong emotions can cause either strong vagal or strong sympathetic stimulation. The former may cause distinct slowing of the heart rate and "blacking out," and the latter may stimulate a rapid, forceful heart rate. Normally we are unable to increase or slow our heart rate by thinking about it. However, a few authentic records have been reported of people who have had this ability.

In an otherwise normal heart, destruction of the SA node, AV node, or the conduction pathway between the atria and ventricles does not necessarily impair the individual's ability to lead an ordinary life. Therefore, medical terms such as complete heart block, AV conduction delay, and bundle branch block describe types of arrhythmias, not actual prognosis. Diphtheria, a disease of early childhood, may cause complete heart block, and coronary artery disease, which occurs so frequently in later life, often produces these arrhythmias. Sometimes these disorders are discovered only during a routine physical checkup in which an electrocardiogram has been taken. Often the patient does not have any complaints referable to the heart and has been living a normal life. There is no reason, under such circumstances, for him to alter his way of living. In fact, much harm can be instigated by alarming the person with discussion of these heart conditions.

ECTOPIC HEARTBEATS

Another striking difference between heart muscle and the other two forms of muscles found in man is that heart muscle cannot be forced to remain contracted. The heart muscle acts on an all-or-none basis. For example, after a stroke of the left ventricle, it cannot be forced to contract again for a short time. This is called the absolute refractory period. This stage is followed by the relative refractory phase in which much stronger stimuli are needed to induce a contraction. After the absolute and relative refractory cycles, a supernormal excitatory phase develops, in which the heart is relatively more susceptible to extraneous stimulation. Presumably during this time excitants, such as excessive alcohol ingestion, tea, coffee, cigarette smoking, and fatigue, may cause premature heartbeats. Apparently a small segment of atrial or ventricular muscle becomes "irritable"; similarly fatigued skeletal muscle may produce twitching. Electrocardiograms reveal that, in most instances, the ectopic beats arise from one focus and more often from a ventricle than from an atrium. These ectopic beats are not signs of organic heart disease. They are universally found in people over thirty years of age, and most people are unaware of them. To some persons, however, the symptoms are distressing, but removal of the offending agent, which is usually cigarettes or coffee, will stop the ectopic beats.

Often the sufferer is afraid that the ectopic beats are caused by coronary artery disease. The physician can reassure the patient by demonstrating that the extrasystoles disappear during exercise. If the person has coronary artery disease, exercise will not only fail to abolish the extrasystoles, but it may even increase them.

TREATMENT OF ARRHYTHMIAS

When arrhythmias are caused by organic heart disease, the doctor has at his command various kinds of antifibrillatory agents, such as quinidine, procaine amide, and digitalis preparations, especially quinidine, which is the most effective antifibrillatory agent, and which acts by soothing the heart muscle when given in small doses. When the dose is increased, the competence of the heart muscle to contract diminishes, and if the use of the drug is intensified, dangerous symptoms and signs appear. In general, the therapeutic and toxic effects of all antifibrillatory drugs are similar. Digitalis preparations act differently. By improving cardiac output and thereby the blood supply to the heart, they may eliminate the arrhythmia. Another course, which may eradicate or lessen the effect of an arrhythmia, is to increase vagal stimulation of the heart. By the latter method, certain types of arrhythmias that produce fast heart rates may be abolished or slowed to relatively normal rates. Singly, or in combination, digitalis and quinidine can inhibit or control all cardiac arrhythmias.

METABOLISM OF THE HEART

Until recently, inquiry into the metabolism of the human heart was impossible. Calculated guesses have been made by studying experiments with animals and by examining respiration of muscle in special apparatus. In the last twenty years intrepid researchers have proved that catheters may be inserted with relative impunity into the chambers of the human heart of a normal person. The nitrous oxide method to determine cerebral circulation was adapted to ascertain coronary artery circulation in dog and man. The coronary sinus, a little opening into the right atrium, drains venous blood chiefly from the left ventricle. With the aid of a catheter inserted into the coronary sinus and the nitrous oxide method, the investigator can determine various fractions of the blood, including oxygen, sugar, fat, and protein drained from the left ventricle. With a simultaneous sampling of arterial blood, both blood flow and metabolism of the left ventricle can be determined.

These conclusions have dispelled some misconceptions concerning metabolism of the heart muscle. The resting heart consumes more oxygen than was previously believed. Following this observation, that the heart muscle of a person at rest consumes increased oxygen, research and study have shown that the differences of the consumption of oxygen between the working and resting heart decrease and indicate that the heart is a much more efficient organ in producing useful energy than was previously surmised. Although it was known that the blood emerging from the coronary sinus was darker than that from other veins because of diminished oxygen, exact measurements show that the heart muscle consumes, per unit of blood passing through it, far more oxygen than any other organ or tissue in the human body. An unexpected discovery is that fatty acids contribute much more to the energy of heart muscle metabolism than does sugar in the form of glucose or lactate.

At present, the blood flow through the coronary arteries to the heart muscle is considered to be proportional to the energy requirements of the heart and not to specific constriction or dilatation due to nervous influences. Studies of metabolism of the heart in congestive heart failure and in diabetes mellitus have revealed little variance from that of normal metabolism. Therefore, apparently the heart not only uses many types of fuel to produce energy but also extracts more oxygen per unit of blood than any other tissue, and its blood flow is proportional to its oxygen requirements.

ADAPTABILITY OF THE HEART

One of the most reassuring things about the heart is its ability to adapt. With normal blood supply, the normal heart muscle cannot be injured permanently by acute or prolonged, severe exertion. The reverse seems to be true. Present studies tend to indicate that people who exercise regularly all their lives suffer from less heart disorders and live longer than their sedentary companions. A London bus driver does not live as long as his active co-worker at the rear end who runs up and down collecting the fares, and "athlete's heart" has been shown to be a myth.

Adaptation of athlete's heart to daily strenuous exercise is somewhat analogous to the recognized ability of a person with a complete heart block to live a full normal life. The person who does not exercise regularly but who indulges spasmodically in strenuous exercise is aware of his fast heart rate and panting respirations. Intensive exercise usually demands an oxygen consumption of five to ten times that of the resting level. The untrained person increases the blood flow to the working muscles by accelerating the heart rate excessively and, actually, by slightly decreasing the output per beat of the heart. The trained, superbly conditioned athlete has a heart muscle approximately the same size as that of the untrained person, but his response is quite different. The disciplined man will have a heart rate at rest considerably under 60 beats and occasionally as low as 40 beats per minute. He will not only be able to do the same work more efficiently, due to factors influenced by training outside of the heart, but also more effectively from the heart action itself. While the untrained person's heart rate speeds from 70 to 120–150 per minute at rest, the trained athlete's heart rate during the same oxygen consumption will rise to 80–100 and the individual stroke output will increase rather than decrease. In other words, the heart of a trained person during the resting period can fill much more completely, and during contraction it can empty more thoroughly than that of the untrained man. As a result, the actual heart rate is much slower.

Current investigations apparently prove that lifelong moderate regular exercise decreases the incidence of coronary artery disease. Therefore a normal person should exercise regularly, not only to keep up general muscle tone but to increase heart muscle efficiency and reserve. He then in all probability will feel better, and he may even live much longer.

EXERCISE AND HEART SIZE

Two of the reasons responsible for the earlier misconceptions concerning the effects of exercise were the apparent enlargement of the borders of the heart in the athlete seen during fluoroscopic examination and the fact that occasionally athletes, or more often former athletes, drop dead. The mistaken diagnosis of enlarged or hypertrophied heart during fluoroscopic examination was due to the ability of the athlete's ventricles to expand more than those of the sedentary individual. Moreover, the hearts of such athletes who have died from accidental causes have been found to be normal. The sudden death of an apparently normal athlete indicates that probably he did not have a thorough medical examination. Such instances are rare now, because all athletes indulging in strenuous exercises are given complete physical examinations including chest films.

In the case of former athletes who drop dead, the most likely cause is unsuspected coronary artery disease, which caused scarring of the heart muscle. A typical illustration is a person who has indulged in little or no exercise for several years, who has become overweight, and who most likely has overindulged in alcoholic beverages and smoking. Such an individual decides that he can still do what he was able to do when he was lighter and in good form. Such tragedies could be avoided by slow, cautious weight reduction, moderation in other habits, and by moderate and gradual resumption of athletic endeavors.

In organic disease that affects the heart, such as defects in the blood vessels, heart valves, and high blood pressure, it must be remembered the heart muscle may hypertrophy, or increase in size and weight. In such instances, hypertrophy of the cardiac muscle is the only compensation possible for the heart. The degree of hypertrophy depends chiefly on the severity of the disorder or disease that puts a strain upon the heart muscle and the condition of the coronary arteries. The ability of the heart with normal coronary arteries to compensate by hypertrophy is amazing. At autopsy, some hearts have been found to weigh almost three times the normal weight—900 grams (nearly 2 pounds) compared with 300 (about 10 ounces). In these instances, hypertrophy is the only way that the heart can compensate for the defect. When the source is eliminated, the heart fibers return to normal size.

Adversely, the heart can become small, or atrophied, when the patient is languishing from cancer or some other disorder or disease that keeps him immobilized for long periods of time. Such a heart can be recognized during life by the small shadow in the X-ray film and at post-mortem examination by the brown discoloration and increased pigment known as brown atrophy. To a certain extent, this shrinking and decreased metabolism of the wasting heart muscle explains the weakness and inertia in the extraordinary increase in heart rate at the slightest exertion. In studies made on normal young adults, such deterioration may explain the observations made during and after prolonged immobilization. These findings consist of increased heart rate, decreased stroke output, and a long delay in regaining normal tolerance to exercise. Furthermore, this seems to be a reversible condition.

INFECTIONS AND THE HEART MUSCLE

Heart muscle is relatively less affected by infectious disease than other organs. In fact, one can count on the fingers of both hands diseases that cause permanent serious changes in heart muscle or death by primarily affecting heart muscle. Certain strains of streptococci produce rheumatic fever, which may cause death within a few days by direct effect upon the heart muscle. Fortunately, this is rare. (Rheumatic fever is discussed in another chapter of this book.) Diphtheria, a completely preventable disease, can leave small residual scars in the heart. The scarring is not significant unless it disturbs the conduction system. A few rare collagen diseases affect the heart in a manner similar to that of rheumatic fever. A few viruses may affect heart muscle principally so that the patient either dies immediately or passes into slow progressive congestive heart failure.

Another rare condition is amyloidosis, which may be primary or more generally due to chronic infection. Seeping of a proteinlike, waxy substance occurs around the muscle cells. Amyloidosis can be diagnosed only by appropriate staining methods at death or by injection of effective dyes during life, if other organs are also involved. The cause of isolated cardiac amyloidosis is unknown. Systemic amyloidosis is due to chronic infections such as bed sores in paraplegics, or persons paralyzed from the waist down. In these cases, preventive measures or prompt therapy can prevent or delay the onset of amyloidosis.

DIRECT BLOWS TO THE CHEST

Formerly the heart muscle was thought to be relatively immune to bruising from blows upon the external chest. Now we know that severe sharp blows delivered to the precordium may cause actual injury despite the fact that the heart is, in most instances, well protected by a bony cage and that it hangs freely in the mediastinum about one-third of the way from the anterior chest to the backbone. The most common types of blows are a violent fall against an inanimate object such as a rock or a piece of wood, a kick by a horse, or the injury caused by striking the chest against the steering wheel in an automobile accident. Anyone subjected to a blow severe enough to "knock out his wind" should be checked by a physician for myocardial damage and should have an electrocardiogram taken. Usually a few days of rest will restore normal heart rate and action. The bruising is generally superficial and the resultant scarring does not permanently affect the heart. Any person stabbed accidentally or on purpose by a sharp object, such as an ice pick, scissors blade, or knife, should be examined immediately by a physician and probably kept under observation for a day or two, so that he is certain that the object did not penetrate to the heart muscle or nick a coronary blood vessel.

HEART MUSCLE AND TOXIC FACTORS

Few poisonous factors have a specific effect upon heart muscle. As has already been explained, therapeutic agents such as digitalis or quinidine can be toxic as well as therapeutic. Emetine, a drug employed to eradicate certain forms of amebic infestation, is another cardiac poison. Since emetine can cause necrosis of heart muscle, the patient must be carefully observed prior to and during treatment with the aid of serial examinations of the heart and electrocardiogram. Although preparations of digitalis have been suspected of causing permanent scarring of the heart, this has never definitely been proved in man. The toxic changes are usually reversible and preventable by slow and careful administration of the drug. This situation is fortunate since the only drug that specifically restores contractibility toward normal in congestive heart failure is digitalis, which produces increased contraction of heart muscle. If digitalis is given in customary doses mistakenly to a person with a normal heart, heart performance not only does not improve, but work tolerance actually decreases. It may change the form of the electrocardiogram and give a false positive reading for coronary artery disease. Its therapeutic action in the failing heart is achieved by shortening the overstretched muscle to normal size and by returning the feebly beating heart muscle to normal contractions.

Metabolic imbalance of the electrolytes of the blood may in themselves cause derangement of the conduction of the specialized neuromuscular tissue. Changes in the sodium, potassium, magnesium, calcium, chloride, phosphate, and bicarbonate of the serum may produce toxicity by enhancing the action of some of the therapeutic agents. For instance, calcium augments the action of digitalis as does a decrease in the potassium blood level. Such changes are thought to be completely reversible by restoring the normal ratio and amounts of these blood constituents. This chapter does not discuss the many and diverse factors that can produce these disturbances in electrolyte balance; whole texts have been written on the subject. These complications interfere with transport of sodium and potassium across the cell membrane, which in turn affects muscular contraction and conduction of the electrical impulses through the heart.

METABOLIC DISORDERS AND THE HEART

Finally, metabolic disorders and diseases may affect heart muscle, but usually to a lesser degree than other organs. Giants and acromegalics often have hearts that are disproportionately large. A considerable number of them die from primary heart failure, and the exact reason is unknown. Certain metabolic diseases such as diabetes, hyperthyroidism, and hypothyroidism can damage heart muscle directly and indirectly. The indirect course is ordinarily induced by producing atherosclerotic changes in the coronary heart arteries as well as in other arteries and by waterlogging the heart muscle. Adequate diagnosis and treatment of these diseases will either prevent or slow down such changes. A lack of vitamin B complex, particularly vitamin B_1, better known as thiamin chloride, can interfere with the metabolism of heart muscle and produce congestive heart failure. This condition, though relatively rare in the United States, must be kept in mind since many people, particularly older persons, do not eat well balanced diets.

The heart muscle is a wonderfully efficient and rugged organ. It not only maintains its own rate through specialized cells, but also can survive and enable the person to lead a relatively normal life when certain of these particular conduction areas are removed. The heart muscle is a most efficient and adaptable organ; it is able to extract more oxygen from the blood than any other tissue, and it can utilize and burn fatty acids as well as sugar. Its blood supply through the coronary arteries is automatically adjusted to the energy requirements and it thrives on regular strenuous exercise. This heart muscle is relatively immune to diseases and drugs, and, if scientists could prevent hardening of the arteries and thus prevent a great number of people from being disabled by, or from dying because of, coronary artery disease, the human heart muscle might beat forever.

CHAPTER VI

The Heart Valves

WALTER S. PRIEST, M.D.

FOUR VALVES are in the heart as a whole. The collecting chamber, or auricle, of the right side of the heart receives blood from the veins throughout the body, which has been collected into two large veins emptying into the right auricle. This venous blood is purplish-red and gives the blue color to the veins you can see under your skin. It has comparatively little oxygen and considerable carbon dioxide. The right side of the heart pumps, or forces, this venous blood through the lungs where it gives up its carbon dioxide and takes on oxygen, which changes the dark color to a bright red. The valve which serves as the door between the right auricle and ventricle is the tricuspid valve, so-called because it is composed of three segments, or leaves. The artery leading out of the right ventricle is called the pulmonic artery. The valve which guards the opening of this artery is called the pulmonic valve.

The left side of the heart gets the freshly oxygenated blood to the bodily tissues. Its collecting chamber, or auricle, receives this blood from the lungs by way of three veins. The valve between the left auricle and ventricle is called the mitral valve because it looks like a bishop's miter. It is composed of two leaflets. The large artery leading from the left ventricle is called the aorta and the valve guarding its opening is the aortic valve. This valve and its corresponding one, the pulmonic valve, on the right side of the heart are composed of three leaflets which are shaped like a half moon. These two valves are sometimes called the semilunar, meaning half-moon, valves.

With the separate functions of the two sides of the heart in mind, you can appreciate why there should be no direct connection between the two sides of the heart. If there were, the venous blood with its low oxygen and high carbon-dioxide content would be circulated through the body. This is what happens in certain congenital defects in the heart and is the cause of the "blue" color of the "blue" baby.

HOW THE VALVES OPEN AND CLOSE

Obviously some means must be provided to insure the opening of the heart valves at the proper time. In the case of the mitral and tricuspid valves, this is accomplished by small, cone-shaped muscles about a half-inch in length and the size of a lead pencil in diameter. These muscles are attached to the inside wall of the ventricles. At the tip of these muscular cones are tiny tendons which fan out to the edges of the valve leaflets. These little muscles are called the papillary muscles. At the proper time in each cycle of the heart, these tiny muscles contract and pull the valve leaflets downward and away from each other until they are flat against the inner wall of their respective ventricles, thus permitting free flow of the blood from the auricle to the ventricle. As the ventricles fill with blood, the pressure within these chambers naturally increases. Toward the end of this filling process, the muscular walls of the ventricles begin to contract. This further increases the pressure within these chambers and, at the proper instant, the leaflets of the pulmonic and aortic valves are forced open by this pressure, permitting the blood to flow into the pulmonic artery and the aorta. A fraction of a second before the pulmonic and aortic valves open, the mitral and tricuspid valves snap shut, thus preventing the blood from flowing back into the ventricles. When all the blood in the ventricles has been forced into the pulmonic artery and aorta, and the ventricles begin to relax, the pressure of the blood in the pulmonic artery and aorta is sufficient to close their respective valves. It is not necessary for these valves to have papillary muscles.

The tissue of the valves themselves is the same as that which lines the cavities, or the chambers, of the heart. It is about as thick as household waxed paper and about as transparent. The individual leaflets of the heart valves are delicate. With their constant opening and closing throughout life every time the heart beats, they "take quite a beating." But, in spite of their apparent delicacy, they are tough. Unless they become inflamed as the result of an attack of rheumatic fever early in life or become infected with bacteria in bacterial endocarditis, they retain their delicate structure and ability to close completely throughout life.

CHANGES IN THE VALVES

Sometimes, in elderly people, the normally thin and sharp edges of the valve leaflets are thickened and have a blunt, or rolled, edge.

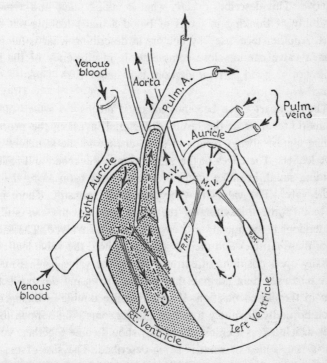

Four valves control the flow of the blood through the heart. In this diagram the arrows indicate the direction of flow through the heart from the right side out through the pulmonic artery to the lungs and back through the pulmonic veins to the left side. The valves are: *T.V.*, tricuspid valve; *P.V.*, pulmonic valve; *A.V.*, aortic valve; *M.V.*, mitral valve. *P.M.* indicates the papillary muscles.

This may prevent the individual leaflets from coming completely together at the time the valve is supposed to be closed. Through the small slit which results, blood may flow back into a chamber. The slight amount of blood which flows backward through such a valve under these conditions rarely, if ever, causes significant impairment in the ability of the heart to function efficiently as a pump. This flowing back of blood has given rise to the term leakage of the heart. This is an unfortunate phrase since it has made some people think of blood leaking outside of the heart. Naturally, such an occurrence would be incompatible with life. Doctors use the term regurgitation in describing such failure of the valves to close completely, with resultant flow-back of blood. This describes exactly what is taking place and avoids the possibility of thinking in terms of blood actually leaking out of the heart. Another term used by doctors in describing what is happening when a valve cannot close completely is insufficiency of the valve. While not as good as regurgitation, it is better than "leakage of the heart."

When a heart valve becomes inflamed during an attack of acute rheumatic fever or as the result of bacterial invasion, the process of healing almost always results in some change in the structure of the valve leaflets. The edges of the valve become thickened and rolled. In addition, small, beadlike lumps of calcium may form along the edges of the valve. The valves may become thick and stiff. There is also apt to be some thickening of the small papillary muscles and their tiny tendons if the mitral, or tricuspid, valve is involved. The shortening of these muscles and their tendons may hold the valve leaflets in a partially open position. In extreme cases, the valve leaflets may become narrower than normal, thus further increasing the gap between them in the closed position. If you visualize double swinging doors, which normally fit snugly together, having something happen to their edges which leaves a crack where they should come together, you will have a rough idea of what is being described. The size of the crack will determine the volume of blood which will flow backward through the valve at the time it is supposed to be tightly closed.

Because the heart is endowed at birth with an enormous amount of reserve capacity for work, a surprising amount of blood can flow backward, or regurgitate, through an incompletely closed valve without seriously interfering with the heart's ability to do its job of pumping an adequate amount of blood through the body or the lungs, as the case may be. So long as the organs and tissues of the body are getting enough blood for their needs, there will be no symptoms of anything being wrong with the heart. In such cases the only way a defective valve can be detected is by listening with a stethoscope over the front of the chest. What is heard is an abnormal sound called a murmur.

MURMURS

When the heart contracts, a sound is produced typically described by pronouncing the syllable "lub." This is called the first heart sound. There is a second sound, shorter and slightly higher pitched, imitated by pronouncing the syllable "dupp." These are the normal heart sounds.

A moving column of fluid always produces a sound. The sound may be too low-pitched for our ears to detect. Thus, as you walk along a fairly broad river, you may not hear the sound of the moving water. But, if you come to an indentation in the bank, which causes the water to swirl around, you can hear a swishing, or murmuring, sound. This swirling of the water is called an eddy, or eddy current. When the blood inside the heart is moving normally from one chamber to another or from a chamber to one of the great arteries, the sound of this movement cannot be detected by our ears. But, if something happens to produce eddy currents, such as occurs when some blood flows backward through an incompletely closed valve, or the blood has to be forced through a narrowed, or incompletely opened, valve, a swishing, or murmuring, sound is produced which can be heard. Sometimes this murmur can be heard by applying the ear directly to the chest wall. Today doctors use a stethoscope in listening to the heart. This instrument shuts out outside noises and enables the doctor to hear murmurs which he could not hear with the naked ear.

Remember that the mere *presence* of a murmur does not, of itself, mean serious heart trouble. A small per cent of murmurs is caused by conditions other than structural damage to the heart and/or its valves.

For example, a heart murmur may be heard in a person who is anemic. When the anemia is corrected, the murmur disappears. Heart murmurs may be heard in many young children who do not have congenital malformation of the heart and who have never had rheumatic fever or other infectious diseases which may damage the heart valves. As the child grows, the murmur disappears.

An interesting example of this occurred in the early years of my twin boys. At the age of three, one of them had what was thought to be a mild case of acute rheumatic fever. Because of the mildness, we were never absolutely sure of the diagnosis, but since a heart murmur appeared he was closely watched during the succeeding months. There being no other signs of damage to his heart, he was permitted to live a normal life. Periodically I would listen to his heart when he was ready for bed. One evening, about a year after the supposed attack of rheumatic fever, and after I had listened to his heart, his twin said, "Daddy, why don't you ever listen to my heart?" Hastening to correct this gross negligence, I listened and heard a murmur as nearly identical to that of the suspect child as two murmurs could possibly be. The second twin had never had anything which could conceivably result in a damaged heart valve. As time went on, the murmur disappeared from both boys. Today they are both husky athletes in their late teens. By all methods of examination at our command today, the suspect boy has a normal heart. Until the murmur of the suspect boy disappeared, we were forced to consider it as indication of *some* structural damage to a valve (the mitral valve in this case). This, however, was not the important point. The *only* important point was that as time went on it became plainly apparent that whatever damage to the valve there was, and whatever the amount of blood regurgitated from one chamber to another by reason of the damaged valve failing to close completely, significant impairment of the heart as a *functioning pump* was absent. Therefore, the child was able to grow and develop normally and to lead as active a life as any of his contemporaries. It would have been a grave mistake to have restricted, or pampered, this child in any way *merely* because he had a heart murmur which had to be considered as evidence of a damaged valve at the time.

ORGANIC AND INNOCENT MURMURS

Doctors often refer to a murmur which they believe to be caused by a damaged heart valve as an organic murmur. The term functional has been applied to a murmur heard in a child who is known not to have a congenital malformation of the heart and who has not had infectious disease which could damage a heart valve. The murmur of the nonsuspect twin in the illustration cited is an example of a functional murmur. A growing, and proper, tendency is avoidance of the word "functional," with classification of murmurs as organic or innocent, the latter term implying that we may not be sure whether a given murmur is the result of a damaged valve or not. But, what we are sure of is that, valve damage or not, the heart is not being impaired in doing its job as a pump, nor is it likely to be. Experience enables us to go even further and to state that there are many, many hearts which acquire damaged valves as the result of some infection and whose murmur or murmurs persist throughout life, without the heart ever failing to do an adequately efficient job as a pump.

MITRAL STENOSIS

So far we have talked about heart valve damage which results in the failure of the valve to close completely. Sometimes, as the result of rheumatic fever, a sticking together of the valve leaflets occurs, which prevents opening all the way when the valve should. This is called stenosis, which means narrowing or stricture. It may not develop until many months, or years, after the acute attack of rheumatic fever. When it does, it tends to become progressively more severe until only a tiny slit, or hole is present when the valve is supposed to be wide open. The valve most commonly involved in this process is the mitral valve, the one between the left auricle and ventricle. For a while, often for years, significant impairment of the heart's function as a pump is absent. As the opening narrows, however, all the blood in the auricle does not have time to flow into the ventricle. The auricle tries to contract harder to force all its blood through the narrowed opening, but cannot quite do it, so some blood remains in the auricle when it should be empty to receive a full load of blood from the lungs.

To take care of this additional burden, the auricle enlarges. At the same time the pressure inside the auricle rises. In time this increased pressure is transmitted backward through the blood vessels of the lungs until its effect is to raise the pressure in the pulmonic artery which carries the blood from the right ventricle to the lungs. In time the pressure in the right ventricle itself rises. Normally it requires much less force to pump the blood through the lungs than it does through the rest of the body. Hence, the muscular wall of the right ventricle is much thinner than that of the left. But, as the resistance in the lungs goes up in stenosis of the mitral valve, the right ventricle has to work harder and harder, and its wall becomes thicker. Finally, it can no longer meet the demands of increased work, and the increased pressure goes all the way back through the right auricle and into the entire venous system of the body. At this point the liver becomes swollen and tender and the ankles and legs begin to swell.

Long before this happens, however, a person with mitral stenosis will have symptoms characteristic of the trouble. Because the left ventricle is not getting the normal amount of blood to pump through the body, the various organs cannot get enough nourishment and the person notices that he tires more quickly than he used to with the same amount of effort. He may not think too much of this. He may even take vitamins to "pep him up." But before long he either notices that he is puffing on climbing an ordinary flight of stairs, or he may waken during the night with the feeling that he isn't getting enough air. This shortness of breath may come as a severe paroxysm which makes him cough and sit up in bed. He may even cough up some bright blood-tinged mucus from his lungs.

These symptoms of mitral stenosis are described in some detail because today it is the one acquired heart valve trouble which is most successfully relieved by surgery. The earlier the opportunity to relieve mitral stenosis surgically, the better chance to restore useful function. Mitral stenosis is usually accompanied by some degree of regurgitation. The effect of this, as well as the presence of other damaged valves in determining whether a worthwhile result can be expected from surgery, is discussed in greater detail in another chapter. Here again the mere presence of a murmur indicating mitral stenosis does not mean that the heart is significantly hampered in performing its job as a pump. Some cases of mitral stenosis seem to progress just so far and then remain, for the rest of a normal life expectancy, at a point which is compatible with an active, symptom-free life. Only your physician can tell how significant the stenosis, or any valve damage, is in terms of reduced efficiency of the heart.

The point should be made here, as it is in other chapters dealing with other forms of heart trouble, that a heart with a damaged valve, or valves, may still be quite adequate for an occupation involving a minimum of physical effort but inadequate for an occupation requiring strenuous physical activity. In some cases changing jobs is the most important thing to be done in prolonging life. At first this may seem an impossibility. But, over the years, I have been impressed by the number of times my patients have been able to do this successfully, once the initial panic of having to face the necessity is gone.

AORTIC VALVE DAMAGE

The aortic valve is the second in frequency of damage as the result of rheumatic fever. As in the case of the mitral valve, the damage may result in either failure of the valve to close completely with resulting regurgitation of blood from the aorta into the left ventricle. Or, the valve leaflets may become glued together with resulting stenosis. Again, both stenosis and regurgitation may be present together. Because the left ventricle is the most powerful of all the chambers of the heart, it is better able to withstand the additional burden of having to cope with the amount of regurgitated blood in addition to that normally coming into it from the left auricle, or the additional force necessary to push the blood through a narrowed opening. Thus it is possible to have certain degrees of regurgitation and/or stenosis of the aortic valve present throughout life without the heart going into failure.

The degree of damage in the aortic valve is more apt to be severe than is the case with the mitral valve. It may be that the terrific force with which the jet of blood strikes this valve when the left ventricle contracts is a factor. If regurgitation predominates, the pressure in the aorta and immediate arteries coming off the aorta may be high at the time of contraction of the left ventricle. But when the ventricle relaxes, the "bottom drops out of the pressure," so to speak. We may see the effect of this in the marked pulsation of the large arteries of the neck. As we get further out in the circulation, we can see an ebb and flow in the movement of the blood. This does not make for efficient nourishing of the tissues. Here again, easy fatigue may be noted as a result.

A more striking effect is noted when stenosis of the aortic valve predominates. Here the blood pressure in the arteries is low. The pulse at the wrist, instead of being "full" and easily felt, is weak and seems to crawl against the finger instead of hitting it. The effect of this is most noticeable in the brain and patients with predominant, or severe, aortic stenosis are subject to fainting spells, especially when they are in the upright position. Fortunately, these extreme degrees of damage to the aortic valve are rare.

For some reason not clearly understood, the valves on the right side of the heart, the tricuspid and pulmonic, are seldom damaged by rheumatic fever. When they are, it is almost always in combination with one or both valves on the left side of the heart. Such multiple valve damage causes serious impairment of the efficiency of the heart, and such patients are apt to be real "heart cripples." Fortunately, such multiple valve damage is extremely rare.

Stenosis of the pulmonic or aortic valve may occur as a congenital defect. The condition is more common in the pulmonic than in the aortic valve. Surgery offers an excellent chance for relief of pulmonic stenosis. Surgery of the aortic valve has not yet reached the same degree of promise. But, with the rapid strides being made in new methods, there is every reason to hope that this will change in the near future. Just as in the case of acquired stenosis of the heart valves, a congenital stenosis does not necessarily mean a severely crippled heart. Sometimes the degree of stenosis of the pulmonic valve is so slight that the risk of operation would not be justified. The author has, among his patients, three adults, two in their fifties and one past sixty, who have congenital aortic stenosis. Yet, their hearts have never failed them and they have lived useful, productive lives.

Just as the failure of a valve to close completely when it should produces eddy currents in the flow of blood which cause a murmur, so does stenosis of a valve. The timing of these murmurs in the heart cycle is different from that of the regurgitant murmur.

A physician is usually able to detect a damaged heart valve by a careful physical examination alone, and, in most instances he can tell which valve (or valves) is involved and whether regurgitation or stenosis, or both, is present. With a complete history from childhood on, and analysis of current symptoms, if any, he can get quite an accurate idea as to how much the valve defect is interfering with the efficiency of the heart as a pump. He may employ certain of the laboratory tests detailed in other chapters as checks on his impressions gained from the history and physical examination. Sometimes he may be in doubt as to just how much a valve defect is reducing the efficiency of the heart, or whether what he hears is caused by an acquired or congenital defect. In this case he may refer you to a heart center for catheterization. Occasionally he may want the opinion of a specialist in heart diseases. If he does, don't get the idea that your condition is serious. Rather, be thankful that you have a physician with a well-developed sense of responsibility who goes all out to render the best possible service to his patients.

ANXIETY AND HEART MURMURS

Consciously, or unconsciously, all of us think of the heart as the most vital organ in our bodies. It is not surprising, therefore, that an anxiety reaction always attends the awareness of heart trouble. The anxiety may *of itself* cause symptoms exactly like those of reduced efficiency of the heart. These symptoms may appear abruptly after the patient is told he has a heart murmur, previously unknown to him.

A few years ago I saw a young woman who, a few weeks after being told she had mitral stenosis, began to complain of easy fatigue, became short of breath on exertion previously well tolerated, and had bouts of severe shortness of breath and cough at night. Prior to the knowledge of her heart trouble she had had none of these symptoms. She was admitted to the hospital for surgical relief of her mitral stenosis. As I watched her and listened to her story, I became suspicious and requested catheterization of her heart. It was shown that the degree of stenosis of her valve was not severe enough to account for her symptoms and that surgery could not have given her any better opening of her valve than she had. Psychologic studies revealed an intense anxiety over the *fact* of anything being wrong with her heart and the threat to her mode of life that "heart trouble" must certainly be. With better understanding of herself, and better insight into the significance of her heart trouble, her symptoms disappeared.

Four years later the stenosis of her valve *had* reached the point where surgical relief was indicated. But, by then she was ready psychologically to get the full benefit from the operation. Had she been operated on earlier, not only would the operation have done her little or no good, I doubt if her symptoms would have been relieved because her basic anxiety would have remained.

PREVENTION OF VALVE DAMAGE

There is no drug which can change the condition of a heart valve once it has become scarred as the result of rheumatic fever or bacterial infection. But we do have, today, methods of treating acute rheumatic fever which we think lessens the severity of the attack and thereby minimizes valve damage. We may even have within our grasp means of preventing the first attack of rheumatic fever. Certainly we do have a proven method for preventing subsequent acute attacks. The antibiotics, especially penicillin, enable us to cure at least 85 per cent of the bacterial infections of the heart valves if we can get to them in time. Until 1944 this condition was practically 100 per cent fatal.

A new development in the early detection of valvular heart trouble is the mass tape recording of heart sounds of school children. This "screening" program was started four years ago as a public service of the Chicago Heart Association. At present it is a combined effort of the Chicago Heart Association, the Chicago Health Department, the

Chicago Board of Education, and the United States Public Health Service. About five out of every thousand children so screened are found to have conditions which justify a detailed heart examination. Few of these have turned out to be serious. Some previously unknown congenital defects which can and should be corrected surgically have been found. The knowledge that a child has a heart valve condition makes it possible to surround him with all the protection and guidance and preventive measures known to modern medicine and at the same time not treat him as an invalid. Of even greater importance has been the finding of some children who were thought to have heart valve trouble but who actually do not have. It is hoped that, in time, this screening of children for heart trouble will become as nation-wide as chest X-ray screening for tuberculosis.

In conclusion, I would re-emphasize: The mere fact of a damaged heart valve is not a ticket to invalidism. Many such hearts are capable of taking care of a normal life expectancy with no more attention on the part of the individual or his physician than the dictates of a sane, hygienic life. Another large percentage of such hearts are capable of doing a satisfactory job for life if the individuals modify their activity and rest habits only slightly and remain under the continuing care of their physicians. The harmful effect of some valve conditions can now be significantly reduced by surgery. This leaves only a small percentage in whom the damage is so severe that only a life of semi-invalidism is possible.

But even in actual house confinement, there are opportunities for usefulness, even gainful, if the affected person will only explore them. I cannot resist telling about a woman whom I have come to call St. Josephine. For the ten years I have known her, and long before that, she has had one of the most severely deformed spines I have ever seen, in addition to a chronic heart condition. For a long time she has been confined to a wheel chair. It is now almost impossible for her to walk. Yet throughout all these years she has supported herself by running a telephone answering service, by sewing and other types of handicraft. In addition she has taken part in community services that did not require outside effort. The influence of her character on her community has been more effective than many sermons.

CHAPTER VII

The Supporting Tissue of the Heart

GENE H. STOLLERMAN, M.D.

ALL ORGANS of the body are composed of tissues that are specialized to perform certain functions. These specialized tissues, in turn, must be cemented and bound together and the whole organ must be properly suspended in order to perform its function most efficiently.

The specialized cells of organs are held in shape by tough and elastic fibrous bundles, cemented together by a mucilagenous semi-liquid material, called the ground substance, and interlaced by a network of fine blood vessels which provide nourishment and remove wastes. These "wrapping materials" are called connective tissues.

In addition, many organs that move actively—the heart, lungs, intestines, for example—require freedom of motion and must hang from the walls of the body's cavities. These organs are therefore suspended from the lining of the chest and abdomen by strong, saclike ligaments made of the fibrous and elastic tissues described above.

The saclike ligament by which the heart is suspended in the chest is called the pericardium. In addition, the heart's powerful muscle fibers are firmly bound by interlacing connective tissues through which course a rich supply of the fine blood vessels that provide the large supply of food and oxygen consumed by the hardest working organ of the body. Also, the heart's inner chambers and its valves are lined by a smooth, tough layer of connective tissue, the endocardium.

THE ANATOMY OF THE PERICARDIUM

Perhaps the easiest way to understand the structure of the pericardial sac is to follow its development in the human embryo. Imagine that the cavity of the chest is filled by an inflated paper bag whose top is compressed tightly around the small ball of the growing heart. As the heart grows and enlarges, it pushes into the sac, carrying with it the compressed top of the bag. Thus, the heart invaginates the top of the sac and eventually fills the cavity so that it is now "a bag within a bag." The top of the sac is now folded around the great blood vessels which emerge from the top of the heart.

The end result of the bag-within-a-bag arrangement is that there are *two* layers of the sac covering the heart; the outer layer, or parietal pericardium, and the inner layer, or visceral pericardium. The latter remains firmly attached to the surface of the heart. Between the layers is a thin space, smoothly oiled by body fluids, so that as the heart contracts and relaxes during its beat, the two surfaces glide smoothly over each other. The heart is thus cleverly and firmly suspended in the inner sac and doubly protected by the outer sac.

EFFECT OF DISEASE OF THE PERICARDIUM AND CONNECTIVE TISSUES ON THE FUNCTION OF THE HEART

Disease of the pericardium may result in two major complications which compromise the function of the heart. Injury and inflammation of the layers of the sac often result in an accumulation of fluid that may fill the sac to various degrees. This fluid may be composed of blood, pus, or serum. If such an accumulation is voluminous, the heart is compressed; it has difficulty in expanding to fill up with blood during its normal beat. This results in reduction of its capacity to pump and symptoms of heart failure ensue. In some such instances, the fluid must be removed surgically by needle puncture or operation.

Another result of severe inflammation or injury of the pericardium is the formation of thick scar tissue during the healing process, which pastes together the two layers of the sac and prevents free motion of the heart. If scarring is extensive, the whole heart may be tightly constricted and incapable of relaxing fully between its beats. This, too, leads to symptoms of heart failure and may require correction by surgery.

Inflammation of the surface layers of the heart sometimes spreads directly to the superficial layers of the underlying heart muscle. The irritated muscle may develop irregularities in the rhythm of its beat and the heart's function may be weakened.

Finally, the connective tissues which entwine the muscle bundles of the heart and which line the heart's chambers may become inflamed by a great variety of diseases that involve connective tissues throughout the body. Such involvement may also weaken the action of the muscle bundles of the heart, may produce scars in its walls and lining, and may destroy the fine blood vessels in the wall of the heart that are required to nourish the muscle.

Diseases affecting connective tissues may frequently involve the heart and that "heart disease" is often only a part—a most important part to be sure—of a more general affliction of the entire body.

DISEASES OF THE PERICARDIUM AND THE CONNECTIVE TISSUES

1) Injury. Crushing or penetrating wounds of the chest may bruise or tear the pericardial sac. If bleeding is profuse and the sac becomes filled with blood, it is imperative to relieve the tension to prevent life-threatening compression, called tamponade, of the heart. More often, however, the pericardium is bruised, and like any other tissue may "weep" a serous discharge into the sac. This is not often likely to be copious enough to result in a medical emergency. Healing of bruises of the pericardium is usually uneventful and does not produce very serious complications unless the damage is extensive or unless there is an accumulation of a large amount of bloody fluid that may ultimately cause extensive scarring of the layers of the pericardial sac and consequent constriction of the heart's action.

2) Infection. The pericardium may become infected in two ways: Infections within the chest cavity, usually originating in the lungs and spreading to the sacs, or pleura, that cover the lungs, may also spread to the outer layer of the adjacent pericardium. Or, an infection entering the body through the respiratory tract—nose, throat, and lungs—or through the intestinal or urinary tracts may be carried along by the

circulation of blood and may eventually lodge in the pericardium. Such infections may be due to bacteria or to viruses.

3) Bacterial infection. An example of a bacterial infection that spreads from the lungs is pneumonia due to the pneumococcus organism. This organism usually involves the lungs first but frequently spreads to the pleura, the sacs covering the lungs, and produces pleurisy. Pus accumulates in the chest cavity and, if the collection is extensive, may also produce inflammation or infection of the pericardial sac. Fortunately, this complication is now rather rare because penicillin treatment is so effective against the pneumococcus.

4) Tuberculosis is another example of a bacterial infection that may spread to the pericardium following tuberculous pneumonia and pleurisy. But the tubercle bacillus may also be carried by the blood stream *directly* to the pericardium, and indeed, a pericardial infection may be the first and only sign of tuberculosis. Fortunately, again, several antibiotics such as streptomycin and isoniazide, are very effective against the tubercle bacillus when the infection is diagnosed early in the disease and before there is extensive pus and scarring in the pericardial sac. For this reason, serious complications from tuberculous pericarditis are becoming much rarer than they used to be prior to the discovery of these antibiotics, and before modern public health programs reduced the prevalence of tuberculosis.

Many other bacterial agents can involve the pericardium directly or indirectly in the same fashion as the pneumococcus and the tubercle bacillus. In most instances advances in accurate clinical and bacteriological diagnosis, antibiotic therapy, and surgical treatment of complications have made bacterial infection of the pericardium a less common and less serious problem than it was but a relatively few years ago.

Bacterial infections within the muscular wall of the heart are not common. Occasionally, in overwhelming infections, abscesses within the heart wall occur but these are quite rare.

5) Bacterial endocarditis. Bacterial infection of the lining of the heart, and its valves, is much more common. Bacterial endocarditis occurs most often in hearts whose valves have been scarred and distorted by rheumatic fever. Should bacteria gain entrance to the blood

stream, following operations or injuries, they may lodge on the deformed valves and grow there. Infection of the endocardium also occurs commonly in some forms of congenital heart disease when, again, bacteria infecting the blood stream stick to the inner wall of the heart in the area of certain congenital defects. Such infections, previously uniformly fatal, are now, for the most part, curable by intensive treatment with penicillin and other antibiotics.

6) Viral infection. The pericardium may become acutely inflamed as a result of a variety of virus infections. These illnesses usually start with general symptoms common to influenza or "la grippe" but then produce severe chest pain and shortness of breath due to inflammation of the pericardium. These attacks usually clear quite spontaneously within a few days or weeks and complete recovery is the rule except in rare cases of overwhelming infection.

Such attacks of benign pericarditis have long been suspected to be due to various viral agents, some of which may also cause pneumonia, pleurisy, and inflammation of the chest muscles and diaphragm. One specific agent, the Coxsackie virus, has been isolated already from several patients with this type of pericarditis and it is likely that in the near future other viruses will be isolated also.

The outlook in virus pericarditis is usually good. Important is early, correct diagnosis, because in its early stages virus pericarditis may produce symptoms and signs that are difficult to distinguish from heart attacks due to coronary occlusion, from rheumatic fever, or from tuberculous pleurisy, all of which are much more serious diseases.

RHEUMATIC DISEASES

Often people are puzzled that "rheumatism," a term implying arthritis, or inflammation of the joints, should also be associated so frequently with inflammation of the heart. If one looks upon the rheumatic diseases as an inflammation of the connective tissues of the body, the connection with the heart is less mysterious. The tissues forming the smooth, glistening, well-oiled surfaces of the joints are very similar indeed to those forming the surfaces of the pericardium, the endocardium (the lining of the heart and valves), and the supporting tissues of the heart muscle fibers.

The rheumatic disease which involves the heart most often is called rheumatic fever. Rheumatic fever is a major cause of pericarditis. Almost always, however, the pericarditis of rheumatic fever is also associated with inflammation of the valves and the muscles of the heart, that is, with *all the connective tissues*. When the inflammation of rheumatic fever subsides, scarring of the pericardium is usually not extensive enough to damage the heart. The much more important problem is scarring and deformity of the connective tissues lining the heart, particularly in the heart valves. Deformity of the heart valves by scarring is the most characteristic and important feature of rheumatic heart disease.

Another form of rheumatic disease which commonly involves the heart goes by the long name of systemic lupus erythematosus. "S.L.E.," as it is abbreviated by sophisticated physicians, is much less common than rheumatic fever but it also inflames all of the connective tissues of the body and therefore can, and frequently does, inflame the pericardium and occasionally the lining of the heart and its valves as well.

The most common inflammatory disease of the joints is rheumatoid arthritis. Fortunately it involves the heart much less often and much less seriously than does either rheumatic fever or systemic lupus erythematosus. It is not a significant cause of symptoms or signs of heart disease. By special microscopic study, however, low-grade inflammation of the connective tissue of the heart may be demonstrated in severe cases of rheumatoid arthritis and occasionally this results in a small amount of scarring.

A variety of other connective-tissue diseases that are relatively rare may also affect the heart. An inflammatory disease of the small blood vessels called periarteritis nodosa; a peculiar disease called *scleroderma* in which excess fibrous tissue is deposited in the skin and in certain organs; and an inflammation of skin and muscle called *dermatomyositis*. These conditions, too, may involve the supporting tissues of the heart in their widespread inflammatory process.

In none of the rheumatic diseases is the cause of the inflammation understood. Rheumatic fever is an exception in that it is now clearly known that this disease is a complication of a sore throat due to the streptococcus bacterium. The streptococcus germ is usually gone from the body by the time rheumatic fever begins. The reason for the inflammation, therefore, is not clear. Nor is it known why almost all of us have one or more streptococcal sore throats at some time in our lives but only certain individuals develop rheumatic fever as a complication.

Incomplete as the knowledge about the cause of rheumatic fever may be, much can now be done to prevent repeated attacks of the disease and to reduce its frequency by proper diagnosis and treatment of streptococcus sore throat.

The agents which cause the other forms of rheumatic diseases mentioned are still unknown, and these diseases remain the object of much intensive current investigation. The solution of these mysteries would eliminate a major category of heart disease.

MISCELLANEOUS CONDITIONS

Although infection and rheumatic inflammation constitute the major causes of diseases that involve the supporting tissues of the heart directly, a great variety of diseases obviously can affect these tissues indirectly in various ways. In coronary disease, the closure of a hardened artery by a clot causes the death and disintegration of heart muscle in the area that was supplied by the obstructed vessel. Inflammation occurs around the dead muscle and this may irritate the overlying pericardium thus producing a local patch of pericarditis.

Another form of pericarditis may develop as a terminal complication of kidney failure, so-called uremia. As nitrogenous wastes accumulate and reach high concentration in the blood, the pericardium may become inflamed and ooze a bloody discharge. This almost always indicates that death is imminent.

Finally, one must consider cancer as a miscellaneous cause of pericardial disease. Cancers that have arisen in, or spread to, the lung and the lymph nodes in the chest may extend directly into the adjacent pericardial sac. Or, the cancer tissue may be brought via the blood stream to the supporting tissues of the heart. The effect of cancer tissue spreading through the pericardium is similar to that described in the above discussion on infection; the heart's motion is encroached upon and heart failure eventually ensues. Cancers that actually start in the pericardium and connective tissues of the heart are extremely rare.

SYMPTOMS OF DISEASE OF THE PERICARDIUM AND SUPPORTING TISSUES

In most instances involvement of the pericardium and the supporting tissues of the heart is not painful. In fact, inflammation of the heart's valves and its lining is quite painless. This is one of the reasons why rheumatic fever goes undetected so often. Many patients are astounded to learn, in later life, that they have a heart murmur from a leaking valve scarred by an earlier, "silent" attack of rheumatic fever that involved primarily the lining of the heart.

When the pericardium is painlessly involved, the patient is unaware of the condition unless the heart's function is compromised as described above. Then symptoms of heart failure may occur. Inadequate filling of the heart causes the liver, abdomen, and legs to swell due to congestion of the veins. Similarly, the lungs may become congested producing shortness of breath.

If inflammation of the pericardium is acute, however, chest pain may occur. This pain is usually an ache in the center of the chest which may spread to the shoulders and down the arms. It is often made worse by deep breathing. Changes in position, such as leaning forward or lying supine, may relieve or intensify the pain.

Severe chest pain of acute pericarditis is most common in benign or virus pericarditis whereas some of the most chronic and damaging forms of pericarditis may be painless. One should bear in mind, therefore, that all acute chest pains arising from the heart do not have the same significance. Proper interpretation of the cause requires careful, expert examination.

The heart, while performing a special and unique function, is constructed, in part, of supporting tissues that are similar to those throughout the body. Thus, it is affected by many diseases that involve these tissues.

The proper diagnosis and treatment of heart disease requires careful determination of the specific areas and structures of the heart that are involved, and demands a clear understanding of the extent to which heart involvement is a reflection of a more general systemic disease.

Chapter VIII

Heart Failure

Aldo A. Luisada, M.D.

Heart failure, cardiac failure, and congestive heart failure are terms used synonymously to indicate a condition which may occur in an advanced stage of heart disease. Usually it is easily recognized because the symptoms, or disturbances, and the signs, or significant alterations in the body of the patient, are typical.

CAUSES OF HEART FAILURE

Heart failure generally occurs in an advanced stage of any disease of the heart, any severe and prolonged increase of blood pressure, and some diseases of the kidneys, blood, certain glands, and lungs. The interval between the onset of the disease and the occurrence of heart failure may be brief or prolonged, but frequently it is many years, even scores of years.

The principal diseases that may lead ultimately to heart failure are:

1) Hypertension, which is a permanent increase in the patient's blood pressure. This may be due to a disease of the kidneys that was followed by high blood pressure, in which case the condition is known as secondary hypertension. Or the high blood pressure may be related to a more complex, partly unknown disturbance involving certain glands, the chemistry of the body, and the nervous system, to some extent as the result of emotion; this type of high blood pressure is called essential hypertension. The primary chamber of the left side of the heart, the left ventricle, is submitted to a continuous strain in all of these cases.

2) A lesion, or damage, of the inner lining of the heart, or the en-docardium, which coats the valves of the heart. Damage to one or more of the valves is due generally to rheumatic fever, and is called rheumatic endocarditis. However, damage may also be caused by bac-teria or other foreign agents that invade the body; then the condition is called bacterial endocarditis.

These diseases ordinarily involve the valves of the left side of the heart, either the aortic or the mitral valve. They may cause either in-sufficient closure of the valve and a resultant leak, known as insuf-ficiency, or an opposite condition, a stiffening of the valve with an incomplete opening for a proper flow of blood, called stenosis. The section of the heart that is submitted to strain is either the left ventricle, in insufficiency, or the right, in stenosis. In some cases both ventricles may be involved.

3) An abnormality in the development of the heart and vessels, described as congenital because it evolves during the nine months of life within the womb of the mother or, less commonly, in a few weeks following birth. The congenital abnormality may be characterized by one of these three irregularities: a) the presence of an unusual open-ing between the two halves of the heart, with a resultant mixture of pure and impure blood; b) an unusually small or narrowed blood vessel or valve that cannot open completely, a form of stenosis; c) a complex malformation, which is the combination of several forms of these abnormalities. (The congenital abnormalities are discussed in Dr. Dry's chapter.)

4) A disease of the coronary arteries, the small branches of the blood vessels which bring blood to the flesh of the heart itself. This ailment, coronary heart disease, usually results in the narrowing of one or more of these arteries, and this tends to form a clot which blocks or closes the vessel. Such a closing is termed coronary occlu-sion. The initial cause of coronary heart disease is usually a progressive formation of hard spots in the walls of the arteries, which is called arteriosclerosis. Arteriosclerosis is greatly influenced by the content of certain fats, or lipids, in the blood, which in turn is influenced by the intake, composition, elimination, and utilization by the body of these components in the daily diet. When such a clot forms, a part

of the heart itself is deprived of nourishment and the heart action becomes weaker.

5) A long-lasting, or chronic, disease of the lungs known as pulmonary heart disease, which changes the structure of the lungs and hinders the circulation of the blood through them. A similar disturbance may occur in hunchbacks or persons with other chest deformities.

6) A grave damage to the muscular part of the heart, or the myocardium, due to a foreign agent—virus, bacterium, or parasite—that results in inflammation and scarring of the flesh of the heart, producing a condition called myocarditis.

7) A severe, enduring disturbance of the rhythm of the heart, which causes a rapid, slow, or irregular heartbeat and is known as tachycardia, bradycardia, or arrhythmia.

8) Acute anemia, prolonged malnutrition, deficiency of certain vitamins, and disturbed function of certain glands may also cause a secondary heart disease.

When damage occurs to the heart valves or when communication between the two halves of the heart is abnormal, also when the blood pressure is elevated, the basic disease causes overwork of the heart, which leads to heart failure. Sometimes, if the muscle of the heart is damaged or works in unfavorable conditions, as in anemia, the disease itself may cause heart failure. It should be kept in mind that often two or more causes are present, and that a heart which is fatigued by overwork may also be damaged in its essential part, the heart muscle.

BASIC TYPES OF HEART FAILURE

Two basic types of heart failure have been recognized. The first is called absolute failure and occurs whenever the heart actually decreases its work. In many such instances, the quantity of blood propelled by the heart into the arteries is smaller than in normal persons. This particular type is called low output failure.

The other basic type is called relative failure. It occurs whenever the body requires a more rapid circulation or a higher blood pressure, or when the damage to the valves requires a greater output. The heart may actually work *more* than a normal heart, but the increase in work is less than is required by the body. In this second type, the quantity of blood propelled by the heart is sometimes greater than average, although it is less than the amount necessary to the body. This particular type of relative heart failure is called high output failure.

THE CONCEPT OF CARDIAC RESERVE

Cardiac reserve is that wide margin of possible increase of work which the normal heart has and which enables it to maintain the circulation even during strenuous efforts. A patient with heart disease usually has a decreased reserve because of one or two possible reasons or a combination of these reasons.

1) The heart is already working more than average, because of high blood pressure, damage to the heart valves, or some other irregularity.

2) The flesh of the heart is damaged, so that the chief function of the heart as a pump is less effective. Direct damage to the heart muscle can be caused by inflammation, disturbance of the metabolism, or a disease of the coronary vessels.

In those patients considered to be in the first group, the reserve is diminished because the heart, acting as a pump, is already performing an increased work. Any further increase, such as is required for walking, running, or climbing stairs, may be beyond the capacity of the heart. In the second group, reserve is diminished because the pump is damaged, and it cannot increase its work if muscular exertion or excitement require extra effort.

RIGHT AND LEFT HEART FAILURE

The heart is composed of two halves. The right half receives the blood from the veins of the body and pumps it into the lungs; the left half acquires the blood from the lungs and pumps it into the arteries of the body. In other words, the normal communication between the two sides of the heart is in the blood vessels of the lungs. Long-persisting diseases of the lungs are followed by increased resistance to the flow of blood which the right side of the heart is propelling. The resistance causes a strain, which weakens this part of the heart; this condition is called right heart failure. High blood pressure and diseases of the valves of the left side of the heart provoke a greater work or an overload of this left side. A disease of the coronary arteries may also cause a direct weakening of this part of the heart, and may result in the so-called left heart failure.

In each of these two possibilities, the blood accumulates behind, or upstream of, the weak part of the heart and the condition is called congestion, while the vessels ahead, or downstream, of the weak part suffer from a diminished flow of blood, known as depletion.

As the accumulation of blood is more easily observed than the depletion, the term congestive failure was coined. However, it should be stressed, first, that any failure of one half of the heart is often followed by failure of the other half, and second, that when flow of blood is continuous and more accumulates in one place, less will be available for circulation in other parts.

HOW HEART FAILURE REVEALS ITSELF

Heart failure can be recognized either through the discomfort that it causes the patient or through obvious signs and manifestations.

1) The patient often suffers from shortness of breath, or dyspnea. This may occur following exertion, or when the patient lies down, or often even during the night as a sudden attack of heavy, sometimes noisy breathing. These three forms of dyspnea represent three stages in the severity of the disturbance and are usually explained as the result of accumulation of blood in the vessels of the lungs because of rather severe left heart failure. In some cases, the accumulation of blood is followed by the passing of a part of the liquid portion of the blood, or plasma, through the walls of the fine vessels, or capillaries, of the lungs into the air chambers, or alveoli, of these organs. The plasma, coming in contact with the air, which is kept in motion by the act of breathing, forms a foam, which then reaches the patient's mouth as a pinkish froth and is emitted, at times in great quantity. This par-

ticular condition is known as lung edema or pulmonary edema, meaning fluid in the lung.

One important result of heart failure, which may be observed by the patient himself, is a sharp decrease in the amount of urine, called oliguria. Other revealing symptoms are nervousness, dizziness, weakness, lack of appetite, feeling of fullness in the abdomen, and pounding of the heart in the chest. Each of these distressing disturbances may be caused by other diseases, but the combination of several is typical and quite informative to the physician.

2) Heart failure is revealed to the physician by several signs or manifestations. First, a small, often irregular pulse is noted. Then, a swelling of the veins in the neck and an enlargement of the liver, which can easily be felt in the abdomen, are discernible, as is a bluish tinge in the patient's lips, called cyanosis. In addition, a certain degree of swelling of the skin of the ankles and feet can be noted, which, when pressed deeply with the finger, remains depressed. This condition is known as pitting edema of the lower extremities.

Most of these symptoms are due to right heart failure, which provokes an increase of pressure in the veins and in the liver and indirectly causes the plasma to pass through the walls of the tiniest vessels, or capillaries, of the skin.

Another significant sign is enlargement of the heart itself, a fact which can easily be verified by placing the patient in front of a fluoroscope or, less accurately, by tapping, or percussing, the chest.

ACUTE AND CHRONIC HEART FAILURE

Heart failure may occur in either a sudden, or acute, form or in a slow, long-enduring form, called chronic. The acute type is usually accompanied by a severe drop in blood pressure and may be marked by dizziness or fainting as well as by severe shortness of breath or foaming at the mouth (that is, by lung edema). The chronic form, however, is revealed by the combination of symptoms and signs that have been previously described.

The acute form of heart failure may be due to a sudden heart attack, to a "shut-off" of blood, or occlusion, in a coronary artery, which is followed by immediate damage to a part of the heart and its general weakening. Such failure may also be due to a sudden stopping of the heart, which may follow a severe disturbance of the rhythm, or it may be caused by the untoward effect of certain drugs including some of those used in anesthesia for surgery.

MECHANISM OF CHRONIC HEART FAILURE

The series of events which leads to the complex picture of congestive heart failure has been fairly well recognized in the last twenty years and may be explained as follows:

a) Heart failure seems to decrease either the amount of blood flow or the amount of oxygen received through the blood by a specific part of the brain. As a result, a chemical substance manufactured by the brain pours into the blood stream and can react at a distance, particularly on the adrenal glands, located above the kidneys. This action is increased by that of another chemical which is produced by the pituitary, the gland of the brain that regulates the most important functions of the body.

b) The adrenal glands, spurred by these chemicals, produce other substances that pass into the blood stream and react on the kidneys by causing a decrease in the elimination of salt and water. Hence the decrease in quantity of urine and the changes in its quality.

c) Following this decreased elimination, an increase may be noted in the quantity of the blood circulating in the body due to dilution with water. This causes a swelling of the veins, or the vessels of the lungs, and an enlargement of the heart itself. The latter is further accentuated by weakness of the heart muscle and by contraction, or narrowing, of the small blood vessels of the body, including small arteries and small veins; this contraction of the small vessels tends to shift a large part of the blood toward the large veins, the heart, and the lungs.

This mechanism explains why the large veins and certain organs— the lungs and the liver—are engorged and distended, why the quantity of urine is decreased, why the patient feels weak, and why the heart is large.

As a result of the congestion of the vessels of the lungs, nerve impulses, running like messengers along the nerves, reach the nerve center that regulates respiration and cause the patient to breathe faster. This condition is known medically as dyspnea. As a result of the dilation and overwork of the heart, and possibly other causes such as inflammation, effect of different poisons—either produced by bacteria or by an altered metabolism, the heartbeat often becomes irregular. In addition, early contractions, or extrasystoles, may occur, or a completely disordered action—atrial fibrillation, complete arrhythmia, or even more complex disturbances. This obviously aggravates the condition by creating one of many possible vicious circles: The weaker the heart, the more disordered its action, and the more disordered the action, the more disturbed the circulation, which results again in an inadequate action of the heart. The same is true for the enlargement of the heart: The larger the heart, the less effective and efficient become its contractions, and the weaker they are, the larger the heart becomes.

TREATMENT OF CHRONIC HEART FAILURE

Treatment of heart failure has become rather complex. In all cases where it is possible, the physician endeavors to modify, correct, or remove the primary cause of damage to the heart and vessels. This can be done, first, by undertaking corrective surgery with the aim of closing any abnormal openings or communication between the two halves of the heart or between vessels. Such surgery may include dilating narrow valves, replacing narrow vessels, and even implanting new valves of plastic material in instances of valve leak. Secondly, it is done by endeavoring to shorten the course of acute diseases, which may damage the flesh of the heart, through use of drugs or antibiotics that destroy invading bacteria, or by the use of certain synthetic or natural substances that decrease inflammation whatever the cause. Thirdly, special drugs to re-establish the normal regularity of the heart rhythm, and glandular extracts or vitamins are prescribed, respectively, whenever a glandular disorder or vitamin deficiency is involved. A fourth measure utilizes appropriate treatment for patients suffering from a coronary occlusion, or heart attack. Fifth, whenever blood pressure is extremely high, the physician can attempt to lower it by appropriate measures and with powerful drugs in order to decrease the overload placed on the heart.

In addition to these significant, but sometimes inadequate, treatments, a basic management for heart failure is undertaken.

The most valuable drug used to combat heart failure is digitalis. Digitalis is a plant which contains potent substances that act on the heart. An extract of the leaves or the pure, crystalline substance which is responsible for the effect may be prescribed.

Digitalis is a stimulant of the heart and has several effects. It increases the power of the heart's contractions, slows down the rapid heartbeat and makes it more regular, and decreases the size of the dilated heart. It also promotes the production of urine and decreases the engorgement of the veins and the internal organs. No wonder that the effects of this drug are still unmatched by any other and that its use is so widespread.

After many years of evaluating the effects of digitalis, it has been determined that the drug should be given in a large dose at first, in order to establish a certain depot of the drug in the body. This is followed by progressively smaller doses, and finally by a replacement or maintenance dose every day. Since the exact amount of digitalis remaining in the body cannot be easily ascertained, treatment with digitalis requires a close collaboration between the patient and his doctor, so that the latter may advise changes of dose according to the symptoms and signs that may be present.

Another important group of drugs called diuretics promote the formation of urine without any noticeable effect on the heart. This is particularly significant because the use of diuretics will increase the effect of digitalis, which would not be possible if they were working in a similar manner on the heart. These drugs may even occasionally be used instead of digitalis. Their action tends to decrease the volume of blood, the swelling of the skin, and the congestion of several organs. At the same time, breathing becomes easier and the patient will not require being propped up with pillows and will sleep better.

Numerous remedies are used including oxygen in the most acute cases, sedatives, drugs that dilate the coronary vessels of the heart in the case of coronary heart disease, drugs that lower blood pressure in cases of high blood pressure, drugs that dilate the bronchi if bronchitis or asthma is present, and many others.

Among the measures that are of definite help in preventing heart failure, the *limitation of kitchen salt* at the table and in cooking is paramount. Since one of the immediate steps in the development of heart failure consists of a decrease in the elimination of salt by the kidneys, it is logical that salt restriction may somewhat delay the onset and decrease the severity of heart failure.

The patient must avoid excessive exertion. If he becomes ill because of a cold or any other disease, particularly one accompanied by fever, he should go to bed and seek prompt medical advice.

CHAPTER IX

Psychosomatic Aspects of Heart Disease

EDWARD WEISS, M.D.*

THE BEST WAY to deal with tension is by action, the next best way is by speech, and the least satisfactory is by thought. Sir Charles Sherrington, a great physiologist, provided this basis for an understanding of psychosomatic disorders that has helped explain many aspects of heart trouble. Anxiety causes tension: If people cannot express this tension in words or deeds, then, like steam under pressure, it expresses itself as symptoms. The symptoms represent a disturbance in the way the body functions.

The heart has long been regarded as the seat of the emotions. We have only to think of the universal use of the heart as a symbol of love and of hate in such expressions as "warmhearted" and "loving with all my heart" as opposed to "hardhearted" and "heartless." The heart, however, is also the organ of sudden death. Therefore, since heart disease is the most common as well as the most serious health problem in the United States, little wonder should arise that anxiety should attach itself to this organ.

PSYCHOSOMATIC MEDICINE AND HEART NEUROSIS

In addition to the great number of people who have heart disease, an even larger number of persons have symptoms referred to the heart region by other conditions although they do not have heart disease. They complain of pain in the region of the heart, palpitation, breathlessness, weakness, fatigue. At first, only discomfort is felt in the heart

* Dr. Weiss died of coronary thrombosis shortly after completing this article.

region followed later by the development of other symptoms, particularly fatigue, which can be overwhelming and may lead to complete invalidism.

The suffering of heart neurosis differs from the pain of angina pectoris, associated with coronary artery disease. In most instances the pangs of angina occur with exertion because the thickened coronary arteries are unable to deliver an adequate supply of blood to the heart muscle. Pain of heart neurosis, however, is apt to occur at rest and is likely to be located in the left chest, where the heart is thought to be, rather than beneath the breastbone as with angina. Nevertheless, this distinction does not always hold. In many cases, certainty as to whether the pain is that of heart neurosis or of angina pectoris is difficult.

Palpitation is a frequent symptom in heart neurosis and often prompts a mistaken diagnosis of heart disease. This discomfort can be quite alarming, especially when due to rapid and irregular heart action. Often the patient is aware of "skipped beats," which actually may be harmless. If a patient can accept the doctor's reassurance that these are insignificant and ignore them, he can go about his business and harm will not come to his heart.

Shortness of breath is a common symptom of heart disease. Two special forms occur—shortness of breath on effort, such as walking up a flight of stairs, and attacks of shortness of breath that are apt to come on suddenly during the night, sometimes accompanied by coughing and expectoration of blood-tinged mucus. The latter always indicates advanced heart disease.

The shortness of breath that occurs with heart neurosis is quite different from both of these. This symptom does not have any particular relationship to effort nor is it associated with the mechanism responsible for the shortness of breath that accompanies acute heart failure. The patient frequently describes the symptom as an inability to get an adequate supply of air. Often he places his hand upon his chest and takes a deep breath to demonstrate the feeling. It is as though he were saying, "Doctor, I have a load on my chest." What he fails to add, but might very well say is, "Perhaps I could get rid of that load by talking about my troubles." In other words, this shortness of breath, or sighing respiration as it is called by physicians, is symbolic of the troubles which burden the patient.

Heart murmurs, noises like the sound of a brook, made by the blood flowing through the heart, may be innocuous as well as indications of heart disease. The problem of differentiation often arises in school physical examinations and in the recruiting of young men for military service, as well as in industrial and insurance examinations. The murmur results from rapid heart action caused by tension. A slight murmur, unaccompanied by other evidences of heart disease, is usually insignificant.

Weakness and faintness are symptoms of heart disease that also occur in emotionally unstable persons who do not have heart disease. Sometimes such weak spells or fainting spells permit a chronic invalid to dominate the environment. As often portrayed on stage and screen, a matriarch achieves an invincible position, and wins many arguments, by exploiting a "weak heart." Putting her hand to the breast, throwing her head back and closing her eyes, she becomes the central character of the drama as the warring members of the family come to terms and carry out her orders.

One of the commonest problems is chronic fatigue, often associated with "a tired heart." At first the complaint is of something else, for example, of pain in the heart region, palpitation, and shortness of breath; but as the physician gets to know the patient better, he discovers that the major problem is chronic fatigue. The basis for fatigue, in the absence of organic disease, is emotional conflict, which uses up energy no longer available for work and social purposes. Fatigue may be so pronounced that the person leads a life of complete invalidism. In an effort to discover the cause, much medical investigation and treatment and suspicion may be focused on the heart.

When evidence of heart disease or any other organic disease is lacking, and emotional conflict is suspected, the patient may be told that he is like an automobile running with its brakes on, which explains why he expends so much energy. People readily grasp the idea that they can learn to adjust the brakes by discussing their personal problems rather than by continuing to focus attention upon the heart.

When patients complain of heart symptoms and fatigue, mood disturbances which are often overshadowed by the physical symptoms should be sought. The mood disturbance may be the most significant signpost pointing to the nature of the illness. Mental depression may vary from occasional moodiness to prolonged severe depression that necessitates hospital care. This phase will be more fully elaborated in the discussion of coronary occlusion.

I always ask a patient what he thinks of his illness. People often have extraordinary ideas, derived from reading and talking to neighbors and through medical contacts. Until these concepts are expressed and understood, little progress can be made in understanding or treating heart neurosis.

THE TREATMENT OF HEART NEUROSIS

If we could select our parents and grandparents, perhaps we might prevent cardiac neurosis. This would obliterate the inheritance of a "nervous" gene as well as providing an escape from a "nervous" environment. The atmospheric mood produced by anxious, heart-conscious parents creates the tensions out of which heart neurosis is bred.

Unfortunately the physician can do almost nothing about inheritance and, too often, little about the environment. However, one avoids focusing attention upon the heart in the course of a general physical examination, especially when dealing with patients predisposed to heart neurosis because of the burden of anxiety which they carry. Instead of cautioning rest to such a person, I recommend that the patient "carry on in spite of symptoms."

Patients frequently attribute remarks to physicians that were not made or were not intended as interpreted. Such circumstances indicate the necessity for more discreet caution. Despite this wariness, however, the doctor cannot always prevent the patient from putting words in his mouth. Furthermore, an occasional person is so obsessed with the idea of heart disease and is so intent on finding something in the words that the physician uses or in his manner that will support his conviction of heart disease that little can be done. Such people may require special psychiatric care.

When heart neurosis has already developed, the problem of eradicating the idea of heart disease and re-establishing health becomes more difficult. At times a careful history and a thorough physical examination, including such laboratory studies as are indicated, may be enough to reassure the person that he does not have heart disease. Usually, however, more is required. The patient must be encouraged to talk about his "other troubles" in order to understand his "heart trouble." As the other troubles are discussed, he becomes less preoccupied with his heart trouble. Then, instead of cautioning rest, the doctor recommends that he "carry on in spite of symptoms." As the person learns that his symptoms can be made better rather than worse by the exercise or effort which he has been afraid to take, he builds up his confidence, which mounts in proportion to the degree of accomplishment. But this is only the beginning. He not only must accept the idea that his symptoms are of emotional origin but he must also understand the nature of his emotional problems. Recovery is not always smooth, and when setbacks occur it is often difficult to persuade the worried person to get on with his program once more.

Tranquilizing drugs are often given not only because the doctor wants to help his patient as quickly as possible but also because patients prevail on doctors to prescribe these drugs.

The enthusiasm for tranquilizers has been truly overwhelming. The millions of tablets that have been used give some indication as to the place of tension in our daily lives. Since this tension is so often attached to the heart, many sufferers from cardiac neurosis and heart disease utilize the tranquilizing drugs in an effort to overcome their anxiety.

These drugs do not produce cures. The tranquilizing pills only suppress feelings; they do not change the underlying mechanisms that are responsible for them. Psychotherapy provides a more fundamental answer to neurotic problems. Difficulties in relation with other people arise within the person himself. While we can make efforts to change the environment or temporarily influence attitudes by the use of drugs, we can only hope to bring about permanent benefit when we can change the person.

People with heart neurosis will frequently retire from many of life's activities, circumscribing and impoverishing their lives. "Go home and take it easy" is a frequent piece of advice, but recommending rest to regain health is not the answer to this problem. For illness of emotional origin, this kind of advice is rarely if ever helpful because such people do not get well by resting nor can they run away from themselves on vacation. To rest is often "to stew in their own juices," and while vacation may provide temporary help by removing them from people to whom they are sensitive, just as often it fails to take them away from the problem because they carry the conflict within themselves. True, when people use up energy in emotional conflict, they have less left for social and work purposes. But they must understand that rest does not provide the answer but is rather an effort to solve their problems.

THE EMOTIONS AND HIGH BLOOD PRESSURE

The emotions play a part in hypertension. When we say to a friend who is about to get angry, "Now look out for your blood pressure," we are actually warning him about the danger of losing his temper.

Perhaps not by chance did the word tension become an important part of the term hypertension. Every doctor allows for the emotional element in individual blood pressure readings. Many people never get over being gun-shy of the blood pressure apparatus. As they put out their arm to have the cuff wrapped about it, one can feel their muscles grow taut. Almost invariably the first blood pressure reading is apt to be higher than subsequent ones. A casual blood pressure reading is not generally accepted as correct. As one doctor has remarked, "The best way to lower blood pressure is to take it a second time."

Rest and reassurance play an important part in the medical management of hypertension patients, both in the relief of symptoms and in the reduction of the blood pressure level. There was a time when this comprised our entire approach to the patient with high blood pressure, that is, rest, reassurance, and sedation. What is not so generally recognized, although the observation is an old one, is that the early symptoms of hypertension are often exactly those of neurosis. Recent years have seen great advances in the medical and surgical treatment of hypertension. While these advances have been spectacular, they have had the unfortunate effect of narrowing our focus on the disease to the exclusion of the emotions. Patients with high blood pressure are anxious patients. Their anxiety has some relationship to elevation of the blood pressure. The emotions, therefore, become one of the multiple factors which probably enter into the cause and certainly enter into the treatment of high blood pressure.

THE SYMPTOMS OF HYPERTENSION

Headache and various forms of head discomforts, dizziness, and constipation, as well as pain in the heart region, breathlessness due to sighing respirations, and fatigue often cannot be explained directly on the basis of high blood pressure. They are out of proportion to the disease. When such people are studied from the psychosomatic point of view, much conflict is discovered in their make-up and also an inability to express their tensions of emotional origin. Hence these tensions seek a way out in the circulatory system. Psychic factors, however, are not the only ones of importance in hypertension. They are important because their modification often benefits the patient, even if the level of blood pressure is uninfluenced.

A woman of middle age complained of constant headache and had been told that it was due to her blood pressure. She had had a complete physical study. Although the blood pressure was considerably elevated at the time that I first saw her, it came down almost to normal after a few days of observation in the hospital without medication. This is not an unusual occurrence—just a few days of rest in the hospital brings about a great change in the level of the blood pressure. Her heart was normal in size, the electrocardiogram was normal, and a study of the back of the eye showed normal retinal blood vessels. Examination of the urine was negative and kidney function was within normal limits. The conclusion was that this woman had essential hypertension but without evidence of circulatory disease. The headache was unrelated to the high blood pressure.

I said to her, "You know, high blood pressure is called hypertension in medical language, and sometimes tension is related to hypertension." She thought that over for a moment and answered, "Well,

Doctor, I think I can improve on that formula. In my house it is 'contention—tension—hypertension!' " Then she told me of the role she played as a "buffer" between an irate husband and a lazy son who was in business with his father, and of the constant quarreling between them. Her sympathy was with her son. She was always trying to shield him. In her buffer role she absorbed punishment and finally had to pay the penalty in symptoms.

Martyrlike people often play this buffer role and seem to have a great capacity for absorbing punishment. But eventually the breaking point comes and symptoms appear. This woman's headache was her way of representing her difficult life situation. It was just as though she were saying, "My husband is a headache to me." Indeed he was. He was having an extramarital affair and made no secret about it. He felt that it was indecent to smoke or drink, but the sexual appetites were normal and were to be indulged and no secret was to be made of the fact. By humiliating his wife before her friends he added to her problem. Perhaps as a result of the interviews she gained enough confidence to present her husband with an ultimatum. Contrary to her worst expectations, he agreed to end the extramarital affair. It made a great difference in her life. Thereafter she was well as far as headaches were concerned, though she still had her hypertension. Disappearance of the headache was an indication that the symptom was due to anxiety and not to disease. The anxiety in turn was related to emotional conflict, and the conflict could only be understood by getting to know the patient as a human being and not just as a medical case.

THE INFLUENCE OF THE DOCTOR

Some physicians decry the widespread use of the hypotensive drugs, those which lower blood pressure. These doctors realize how difficult it is to judge blood pressure responses; credit is sometimes given to the drug when it belongs elsewhere. Spontaneous variations occur in the course of the disease. The doctor-patient relationship itself is capable of influencing the level of the blood pressure as well as the symptoms. For example, a patient in the hospital may be taking a drug which should be lowering the blood pressure but he is anxious about some situation at home or resents the attitude of some of the hospital personnel and his blood pressure goes up instead of down.

Symptoms of hypertension usually arise in a social setting of emotional stress. One must always question the relation of the symptoms to the high blood pressure itself and make an effort to understand them from the point of view of behavior. Moreover, with the discovery of the hypertension a "blood pressure phobia" often begins. The person becomes overconcerned about his blood pressure, and this anxiety becomes an important part of his symptoms. The symptoms due to anxiety may be alleviated if the person can be sufficiently reassured. The symptoms are influenced by the confidence that the patient has in his physician and the attitude of the physician toward the illness. If the symptoms disappear while some special drug is being given, the drug gets credit. The same is true of surgery, of which it has sometimes been said, "The symptoms disappeared although the blood pressure was uninfluenced," as though to justify the surgery on the basis that it relieves symptoms. The important question is whether the course of the blood vessel disease that accompanies hypertension has been influenced, because this has most to do with length of life and freedom from the organic complications.

PSYCHOSOMATIC ASPECTS OF TREATMENT

When the doctor explains to patients that tension has something to do with hypertension and that such tension may seek a way out in the circulatory system, a door may open that permits the patient to talk about himself as a person rather than as just a case of high blood pressure. I often say, "You are like a teakettle on the stove; if the steam can't get out the spout, it tries to blow the lid off." Thus, the knowledge that every psychic tendency seeks adequate bodily expression gives a practical hint in dealing with patients who have high blood pressure.

While hypertension in itself is not always an indication for psychotherapy, the emotional problems which occur in association with hypertension are such an indication. They are so common that psychotherapy must be considered for many patients with hypertension. There is no reason why it cannot be combined with medical and surgical treatment.

HEART DISEASE PLUS ANXIETY

Important as anxiety is in relation to the normal heart, it is even more important in organic heart disease. While people with normal hearts who are anxious may make themselves and their families miserable, they can live a normal span of years. But the anxious person with a diseased heart may suffer a premature breakdown because the anxiety imposes a real physiological burden on the overworked heart. Many people could carry on successfully with their diseased hearts if they weren't burdened with these additional problems.

EMOTIONAL FACTORS IN HEART FAILURE

A woman of middle age had been admitted to the hospital on some twenty occasions over a period of six or eight years. She was a large, florid woman of Irish parents. She had mild diabetes and slight elevation of blood pressure and suffered from repeated attacks of heart failure. The attacks occurred in the following fashion. She became nauseated and vomited; then her body began to swell, and shortness of breath increased until hospitalization became necessary. In the hospital the time-honored remedies—morphine and oxygen, digitalis and mercury—proved effective, and in a short time she was much better. She got rid of about twenty or thirty pounds of fluid in a week or two, just as though she were a sponge that had been squeezed dry. She felt quite well again and went home. Within a few weeks or a month or two the process was repeated, and she was back in the hospital.

The reasons why she was so "refractory" to treatment were much discussed in our hospital. Why did she refuse to get well and stay well? The possibility of some unusual complication was considered, but nothing was said about this woman as a person. Did her personal life have anything to do with the illness?

She lived with an only daughter in a tiny apartment near the hospital. The daughter worked at one of the big plants in North Philadelphia. On the daughter's take-home pay of $41 per week the two had to live, and insulin, digitalis, and special food had to be bought for the mother. Since the money was insufficient to cover all the expenses, the mother ran out of medicine, became ill, and had to be brought to the hospital. This appeared to be a fairly plausible explanation, but like so many situations in life that seem so easily explained, if one probes a bit deeper one will find that there is more to the story.

The patient confessed that often, just before she broke down, she had had a fight with her daughter. She became upset, "fed up," and started to "throw up," as though to say, "I can't tolerate this situation." Thus an attack was initiated. Now why did this woman fight with her daughter? Inquiry established that the daughter started the fights with her mother. The daughter, a single girl in her late twenties, was thinking, and sometimes saying, "I have to sacrifice everything for you; you are a millstone around my neck. If I didn't have to spend my hard-earned money on you, I could have clothes, I could have boy friends, I could go out and do the things that the other girls do. But I promised Granny [the patient's mother] on her deathbed that I'd take care of you, and I intend to do it."

Thus this woman lived with the constant reproach of considering herself a burden to her daughter, and felt that her life depended upon a deathbed promise. She was resentful but guilty. Frequently, when she left the hospital feeling fairly well, she went home and kept herself busy doing things around the house to please her daughter. She prepared dishes that the daughter liked, cleaned the house, and performed other chores that she ought not to have done. Soon she was back in the hospital again.

Among many other aspects to this problem, the fights occurred just before the daughter's menstrual periods. The daughter had painful menstruation and suffered from premenstrual tension, becoming irritable and difficult just before her period. At this time she was apt to fight with her mother and say the harsh things which she later regretted; but then it was too late—the mother was in the hospital. Therefore, there was a somatopsychic as well as a psychosomatic problem. In other words, the endocrine balance of the daughter had to be taken into consideration in this involved medico-social problem.

Quite by chance we discovered an important psychological factor. The daughter was illegitimate and knew it, and this was the source of much of her resentment and, of course, of much of the mother's guilt.

Finally, the mother died of heart failure. Even though the autopsy was able to demonstrate the diseased heart, it could not show the illness of the spirit.

CORONARY HEART DISEASE

Many patients with coronary artery disease realize that feelings, as well as effort, may cause pain; for example, anger or sexual excitement. These result in speeding heart action; the heart muscle calls for more blood to nourish it, but the narrowed or roughened coronary vessels are unable to furnish the additional amount of blood. Then the heart muscle cries out in protest with anginal pains. But this process does not lend itself to mathematical formulation. Under certain circumstances pain may occur; and again, under identical circumstances, as far as physical effort is concerned, pain is absent. The difference may be in the feelings and attitudes of the patient. Under stress he may have pain, but when at peace with himself there is no pain, although he may be exerting the same or even greater effort. A man of sixty had pain every morning while walking a short distance to his job, which he hated, but on vacation he could walk miles without pain.

In coronary occlusion the symptoms of the patient and the seriousness of the attack depend on many factors, such as the size of the occluded artery, the suddenness of the closure, the extent of collateral circulation, and the condition of the heart at the time the clot formed. The reaction to the attack, which influences recovery, has much to do with the personality of the patient.

Rest has been the keynote of treatment for coronary occlusion, but this means more than just bodily rest. Patients were often confined to bed with strict precautions against making the slightest movement, while attention was not paid to the emotional tensions that enter so importantly into the healing process. An essential part of treatment is to secure the patient's emotional tranquillity. The doctor must be aware of the patient's attitudes and fears for himself and his family. For some personalities rigid bed rest does more harm than good, and as a consequence the "chair treatment" is recommended for some people. If, for example, a patient frets at immobility, refuses to use a bedpan, and is generally unhappy about being confined, sitting in a chair lessens emotional tension and is less hard on him from a purely physical standpoint. For most people, rest can be enforced and nothing takes its place. Even though the patient may feel better in a few days and wants to be up and about, the rest that leads to the healing of myocardial infarction usually must continue for weeks.

President Eisenhower's recovery had a great deal to do with mitigating the public's fears of a heart attack. The courageous advice of his physicians that permitted him to lead a normal life, including exercise, brought home to the average man that a heart attack doesn't necessarily mean invalidism. On the contrary, complete recovery may occur, permitting one to lead a normal life again.

EMOTIONAL STRESS AND CORONARY DISEASE

Medical observations concerning stress have been focused chiefly on physical exertion. Except for an occasional case report to the effect that coronary thrombosis seems to follow almost immediately after great emotional strain, little has been done to make systematic studies. Actually "stress and strain" are regarded by nonmedical as well as medical people as an integral part of the problem of coronary thrombosis. Our concern with disease rather than disorder, that is, our concentration on changes in organs and tissues brought about by disease processes without a comparable study of personality and life situation, has encouraged us to think of coronary thrombosis as a purely physical disease, with emphasis on heredity, dietary factors, and easily demonstrable coronary atherosclerosis. The frequent onset of coronary thrombosis during sleep or rest has also inclined observers to minimize emotional stress. The thought has been, "How could there be stress or strain if one is asleep or at rest?" Emotional factors have also been neglected in regard to the treatment of coronary thrombosis; physical rest and physical measures have been emphasized.

I would not minimize the pre-existing coronary artery disease that is the essential background for coronary occlusion. However, emotional stress may increase the work of the heart: You have only to note your own increased heart rate during excitement to know that this is so. Changes in the blood pressure, the pulse rate, and in the cardiac output have all been measured before, during, and after emotional stress. The same is true for blood cholesterol; many observers have noted higher levels during periods of stress. Clotting time and the viscosity of the blood may also be influenced by emotional stress, so apparently physiological changes may be brought about that increase the work of the heart and impair its efficiency. Thus emotional factors might conceivably add to the burden of an impaired coronary circulation.

Our own studies of personality and life situation of patients with coronary occlusion show that chronic tension of emotional origin existed prior to the onset of occlusion in almost half of a group of sixty coronary patients. We found no such evidence of chronic tension prior to the onset of illness in a control group who did not have coronary occlusion.

EVIDENCES OF TENSION

Evidence of chronic tension is not always obvious to the observer, nor is it often apparent to the patient. Sometimes members of the family, and especially the spouse, help us in obtaining such information. Increased smoking and drinking, which are sometimes blamed for the coronary occlusion, are often only the evidences of increased tension of nervous origin. The same is true of irritability and suppressed anger, as well as sleeplessness, indecisiveness, withdrawal from social contacts, increased dependency on a spouse, obsessive thinking, preoccupation with bodily symptoms, inability to concentrate, disturbances in memory, impotence, depression, and fear of insanity.

Warning signals are: 1) tension and inability to relax, 2) needing a drink or several drinks to get through the day, 3) poor sleep, 4) the use of tranquilizers and sleeping medicines (or worse yet, sleeping medicine followed by a stimulant to wake one up), 5) developing a dislike for responsibility and becoming reluctant to accept promotion in a job.

A machinist of forty-three was admitted to the hospital following an attack of coronary occlusion. He was prematurely gray, a passive and compulsive person. He had been dominated by his father, also a machinist, toward whom he had been totally submissive, and he had been betrayed by his first wife, who had been unfaithful to him. He was a hard worker, took great pride in the quality of his work, and when he felt that his work was not being appreciated, he was filled with anger which he was unable to express. He felt himself heading for catastrophe. There were signs of mounting tension, such as sleeplessness, disturbances in bowel function, irritability, indecisiveness, difficulty in "getting himself going in the morning," and a lack of interest in sex.

He described the events leading up to the attack as follows: "Everything had been fine at work until the last few weeks. Then they started a speed-up, smashing the equipment and, because of the increased load on the machinery, as fast as we rebuilt it they smashed it again. Work used to be enjoyable but now I hated to get up in the morning. The job got me down. I took my work home with me. Something had to happen. This [pointing to his heart] is the result. I couldn't talk to anybody about it but I am glad to get it off my chest."

At first we had some concern that discussing emotional problems with a sick patient might make him worse. Our apprehensions were relieved when we found that many patients welcomed the opportunity to talk about themselves and apparently derived great benefit from "getting things off their chest." Often a patient who had been put to bed with the enforcement of strict bed rest was full of tension and was greatly relieved by the opportunity of talking about his many problems.

SEXUAL PROBLEMS AND HEART DISEASE

The coronary age is also the age of diminishing potency. Sexual problems creating tension occur, especially among men. Since men are much more likely to have coronary artery disease than women, these tensions are of particular significance. In almost 50 per cent of our coronary cases there were important sexual problems that antedated the attack, and most of these occurred in men. They were twice as frequent in the coronary group as in the control group. Loss of desire, quick ejaculation, a feeling of "growing old," preoccupation with the idea of "loss of manhood" or the onset of the "change of life," and compensatory efforts to prove oneself still a vigorous man (a frequent source of stress and strain)—these are some of the problems that afflict men of this age. As previously mentioned, sexual difficulty is just another indication of chronic tension, but one which is apt to be of greater concern and therefore in itself productive of more tension.

Very often after heart attacks the patient is instructed by his doctor "to take it easy" in regard to sexual intercourse, so that he approaches the act of intercourse with considerable anxiety. The same is true for his wife, who already may feel that she has been in part responsible for her husband's heart attack. In general where marital intercourse takes place in an atmosphere of a good, affectionate relationship with a healthy spouse willing to cooperate, it is helpful rather than harmful to permit it, once the patient has recovered from the acute phase of the illness.

REACTIONS TO HEART ATTACKS

The emotions are involved at every stage of heart disease, from the beginning of the attack through the period of rehabilitation. Delayed recovery is a common problem, and physical factors alone cannot explain why convalescence is so long in some cases and so short in others. Some patients actually never recover. The attack is a crucial turning point in their lives; a state of semi-invalidism is maintained indefinitely; little or no work is done, and former responsibilities are never taken up again.

Remember that regression occurs in all illness. An unconscious urge exists to return to a state of early childhood in which there is no responsibility. The emotional interest of the patient is withdrawn from the outside world and centered on himself. Regression is a part of the picture of depression and may exist as hypochondriacal obsession with heart symptoms. It seems to occur in people with strong passive and dependent character traits which become exaggerated. The patient may become an invalid, sometimes subsisting on insurance benefits. Depending on how the situation is handled by doctors, nurses, and family, recovery can be facilitated or delayed, perhaps indefinitely.

The physician, who is human, wants to appear as a benefactor to his patient. If he emphasizes the seriousness of the illness, recommends prolonged rest, forbids sexual intercourse, and surrounds the patient with special precautions, he often plays into the unconscious desire of the patient to remain ill.

The problem of the diagnosis of chest pain after coronary thrombosis is one of the most difficult in medicine. The situation often depends as much upon an analysis of the personality of the patient as upon an evaluation of his heart and blood vessel disease. The degree of psychological impairment must be determined as carefully as the degree of organic heart damage. In other words, the physician must understand the personality as well as the heart, for both have a structure that can be analyzed in relation to prognosis.

Many difficult questions arise under the best of circumstances, but when there is the added factor of a passive and dependent personality who is willing to exploit the illness for purposes of compensation, the illness becomes difficult to control. The doctor is afraid that if he encourages such patients to become active and another heart attack occurs, he will not be forgiven. Hence he sometimes errs on the side of caution, and permits people to continue with the illness, because in many instances it is difficult to say that pain in the heart region is not due to coronary insufficiency. Aware of the history of a heart attack and perhaps a tendency toward heart attacks in the family, the doctor is fearful that it may happen again. Although many patients with heart neurosis but no heart disease go through life with "heart symptoms" as an excuse for not measuring up to their responsibilities, occasionally a patient who fears heart disease eventually develops the disease. No matter how many years afterward this happens, the doctor who declared the patient free of heart disease and able to carry on is condemned for having missed the diagnosis.

Many a wife won't let her husband recover because she feels an inner sense of guilt—if she hadn't made so many demands on her husband prior to the attack, it would not have occurred. Therefore, she must surround him with all kinds of overprotection and oversolicitous care to make up for the sense of guilt. Even before the attack she may have mothered her husband and made him as dependent as a child, and afterward she hovers over him with anxious concern, waiting upon him hand and foot. The nurse, too, in her efforts to be efficient and helpful, may make the patient so dependent that when she leaves he is without support.

DENIAL OF ILLNESS

Although the majority of patients who have had a coronary attack react normally and eventually make a complete recovery, what may be called denial of illness often occurs. It is common in cancer cases where the patient acknowledges intellectually that he has cancer but behaves as though he did not. The same is true in heart disease and is of even greater significance because denial of illness may lead to self-destructive behavior such as the refusal to accept orders, "forgetting" to take medicine, and unwise behavior in general. Rigid enforcement of restrictions in such patients may cause additional anxiety. The psychological need to deny illness may be so intense that it is actually less harmful to permit some activity than to impose the degree of inactivity which seems indicated on the basis of physical considerations alone. Perhaps this is one of the reasons that the chair treatment has been helpful. There are certain people who cannot stand immobility, and even though physical considerations suggest that it is in order, more tension is created by insisting upon it than by allowing a certain amount of activity, such as sitting in an easy chair or allowing the legs to dangle over the side of the bed. Fifteen per cent of our coronary group exhibited the reaction of denial and in some of these a permissive attitude toward a little activity seemed the best way to deal with the situation.

DEPRESSION

Some degree of depression may be considered a normal reaction in anyone who has suffered a heart attack but as healing occurs, apprehension should diminish and symptoms disappear. A normal mood returns as recovery progresses and the reality of the situation indicates that one can live and work normally again. Not so with depression, however, which occurred in 14 per cent of our group. Here the depressed mood continues and heart symptoms, such as pains in the heart region, palpitation, and fatigue, persist. Sleep is poor, with early morning awakening, there is difficulty in concentrating, memory lapses occur with fear of losing the mind, the sex drive is diminished, fatigue is prominent, and suicidal thoughts are common although not often volunteered. The patient complains of heart symptoms, and only as one gets to know the person in the patient are the other symptoms mentioned. It is important to recognize mental depression because it influences so many important decisions, such as resigning from work, selling a home, and getting a divorce. Then, too, there is the actual danger of suicide.

The patient with mental depression is hard on his family, especially the wife or husband. A man may have seemed independent, ambitious, and capable, but after his heart attack he may be fussy, demanding, irritable, and indecisive. Whereas previously his wife felt that he was somebody whom she could depend upon, now he leans upon her, never wants her to leave his side, and at the same time worries that "he is a burden to her." All the time that he is verbally expressing his concern that he is a nuisance and a burden to his family, he quite obviously makes no effort to change this situation and resents advice "to snap out of it" or to attempt to do things on his own. Those who are near and dear to him find difficulty in suppressing irritation with his behavior. They become impatient with his constant reiteration that he is eager to get well when it is his obvious unconscious determination to remain sick.

Much of his concern surrounds the heart. It is not easy to persuade such a person that he has recovered from his heart attack and is able to return to normal living again. As the patient discusses his other troubles, recovery occurs from the heart trouble. This is done gradually. To present the idea that the illness is largely emotional, without paving the way carefully, is sure to arouse resentment. One cannot go faster than the patient is prepared to go, which means that the process of emotional re-education must be gradual.

X Ray and Electrocardiograph

DAVID SCHERF, M.D.

THE SCIENCE of X rays as they are used in the diagnosis and treatment of disease is called radiology. It is also called roentgenology, after Wilhelm Roentgen, who discovered these rays in 1895.

A characteristic of X rays that makes them especially useful is their ability to penetrate bodily tissues. Different tissues are penetrated to diverse degrees. The massive heart muscle and large vessels, such as the aorta, do not permit much transmission of the rays. However, the lungs surrounding these structures, being comparable to air-filled bubbles, offer little resistance to X rays. These differences permit a contrast image of the organs of the chest to be obtained by the use of X rays.

This image can be seen either directly on a fluoroscope screen or recorded on photographic film, called a radiogram. A radiogram permits study of the image at leisure, as well as comparison with radiograms made at other times. The advantage of fluoroscopy is that the heart in motion can be directly observed. Its disadvantages are that the patient gets a greater exposure to the X rays and that a permanent record is not obtained. The exposure can be minimized by opening the shutter as little as possible and thus working with a small field of vision. The outlines of the heart can be drawn on the fluoroscope screen and copied; this drawing is known as an orthodiagram.

THE SIZE OF THE HEART

Before the introduction of X rays, the size of the heart was determined only by percussing, or thumping, the chest. This is a valuable and useful method when done by an expert, but long practice is essential to develop the skill required to get reliable results. This method cannot always be employed; deformities of the chest wall or abnormalities of the lung may preclude its use. But determination of the size of the heart with X rays is easily made.

In most instances when the heart is either normal or definitely enlarged, the physician can see the condition at a glance on the radiogram, although difficulties and mistakes may occur in borderline cases.

The first difficulty arises because the size of the heart depends upon many factors. The heart, even the perfectly healthy one, of a man with a sedentary occupation not engaged in any sport will be smaller than that of the man engaged in physical labor or in athletics. A higher position of the diaphragm in obese people or those with much gas in the abdomen will rotate a normal heart and make it appear larger. Conversely, a low diaphragm in a tall person may make a slightly enlarged heart appear normal. Since the diaphragm moves up and down with respiration, it is important to know the phase of respiration in which the radiogram is taken.

Just as the shadow of an object varies in size depending upon the distance of the object from the light source, the X-ray image will also vary with the distance of the chest from the X-ray tube. In order to avoid misinterpretation of size, standard practice is to X-ray the chest with the patient at exactly six feet from the X-ray tube. Even so, distortion is not completely avoidable, and in obese patients as well as in patients with a deep chest, the heart appears to be larger than actual, and cardiac enlargement is wrongly diagnosed in healthy persons.

The heart size depends also upon the heart rate. Some people, particularly athletes in excellent physical condition, have slow heart rates. With slow rates, more time is available for the heart to fill with blood between beats; hence the heart becomes more distended and larger. For this reason athletes were often said to have large hearts. However, if physical work is performed in an unreasonable and exaggerated fashion, an abnormal enlargement may occur.

Radiologic interpretations often report a small heart. This is not an abnormality, since a small heart is not the cause of any disease; it indicates only that the heart is not enlarged.

A finding which may frighten a patient unnecessarily is described as a fat pad around the heart. This is a normal accumulation of fat near the tip of the heart, not in the heart itself, but only in its covering.

A patient may live throughout a normal life span without heart trouble, in spite of a large heart. For example, a person might have had diphtheria in his youth, which involved his heart and left some scars. Such a person, after recovery from the acute infection, may not experience any heart trouble although his heart is larger than normal. Another may have had mild rheumatic heart disease which never handicapped him and did not require too great restrictions at any time. Nevertheless the heart adapted itself by slight enlargement of some of its chambers. Conversely, a heart of normal size may be sorely affected. Thus in heart attacks caused by coronary occlusions, the heart may be of normal size in spite of extensive damage to the heart muscle.

THE SHAPE OF THE HEART

X rays permit the physician to see at a glance the shape of the heart. The heart consists of four chambers, and the enlargement of any one of them will cause a characteristic change in the shape of the heart shadow, which will often facilitate the diagnosis.

Determination of the shape of the aorta is usually not difficult with X ray. This largest artery of the body is clearly visible in X-ray examination of the chest, and enlargement of the aorta is readily apparent. The significance of such an enlargement varies. For example, in patients of sixty and over, a moderate enlargement of the aortic knob, or widening of the aorta, is due to a harmless action.

THE MOVEMENTS OF THE HEART

Movements of the heart are particularly informative, and the great advantage of fluoroscopy as compared to radiography consists in being able to watch the heart in motion. One famous radiologist has compared fluoroscopy to a motion picture and radiography to a picture postcard. The quick, jerky action of the heart in a nervous person or in a patient with hyperfunction of the thyroid gland, or the slow or almost invisible movement of the heart borders in a patient with a serious involvement of the heart muscle or with fluid in the pericardial sac, are invaluable observations.

X-ray examination readily permits the detection of calcifications, or bone formation, in the heart muscle. This is not unusual, as calcification of parts of the heart are found in a variety of conditions which may be harmless and do not handicap the patient. They may be compatible with a long and healthy life. A "bone in the heart" is a calcification, normally found in some animal species.

Every examination of the heart also includes an evaluation of the condition of the lung. When heart weakness appears, congestion in the lung is found early and manifested by accumulations of fluid in different portions of lungs. The discovery of pulmonary congestion by X ray may precede any other signs of heart failure for a long time, thus permitting an early initiation of therapy.

NEWER METHODS WITH X RAY

Other improvements have been introduced in the X-ray examination of the heart by the use of new techniques. One of these is the use of image intensifiers in fluoroscopy. With the aid of image intensifiers, the exposure of the patient to X ray during fluoroscopy may be lessened.

Angiocardiography is the injection into the vein of substances opaque to X ray, such as certain iodine preparations. When such substances reach certain portions of the heart, they are outlined more clearly and evaluation of size and form is made easier. Furthermore, in congenital abnormalities of the heart, pathologic connections between cardiac chambers are thus quickly detected. Angiocardiography is a most significant aid in the pre-operative examination of certain heart diseases and also in the detection of narrowing or occlusion of arteries. If the roentgenograms are taken rapidly, a technique called cineangiocardiography, a moving picture of the spread of the dye is possible.

The introduction of a catheter into the heart through an opened vein is now a new invaluable tool for the evaluation of conditions for which cardiac surgery may be indicated. The position of the catheter in the heart is controlled constantly by X rays, and an expert in X-ray examination is always a member of the cardiac team performing the catheterizations. Occasionally an opaque substance is introduced, with the aid of the catheter, directly into certain areas of the heart, and this form of angiocardiography gives considerable information about the situation that the surgeon will encounter when surgical repair seems necessary.

Kymography is the technique of registering the movements of the borders of the heart, with the aid of a simple mechanical device. Fluorokymography, using photoelectric devices, serves a similar purpose.

Rheocardiography measures, with selen cells, the density of the shadow of the heart. In planimetry or tomography, an X-ray plate is taken in different planes, and thereby the heart can be examined at different depths.

THE ELECTROCARDIOGRAM

Like all other muscles and nerves, the heart has electrical activity, and this activity can be measured. The machine used to provide this measurement is the electrocardiograph, and the record obtained is the electrocardiogram.

Contraction of the heart muscle is preceded by excitation. During these episodes, ions, chiefly sodium and potassium, move in and out of the muscle cells. The ionic movement is accompanied by the creation of an electric field. Like a magnetic field, it has a negative and a positive side and may be measured at a distance. When an impulse to contract spreads over the heart, it behaves electrically as small batteries do, moving with the positive and negative poles, or dipoles, close together, the positive in front of the negative pole. About 90 per cent of the potentials thus created neutralize each other, since the activation of the heart proceeds in different directions. An electrical field created by activation of a certain muscle strip in one direction is neutralized by another field caused by the excitation of a muscle strip of the same size running in the opposite direction.

In most cases we can measure, with the electrocardiograph, only the potentials that reach the surface of the body. The electrocardiograph picks up the potentials, magnifies them many hundreds of times, and records them on a strip of paper. This tracing is the electrocardiogram.

By tradition first, and later by convention, these potentials were registered from definite points known as the lead points, to which metal plates, the electrodes, were applied. They pick up different potentials at the lead points and these potential differences are registered. The old electrocardiographs were large and cumbersome because it was necessary to use electromagnets for magnification. Electronic devices have replaced these and make the machines easily portable. The electrocardiographic tracing is written directly on especially prepared paper.

The electrodes are applied after the skin is rubbed with a jelly containing pumice, which serves to diminish the electrical resistance of the skin. At first these lead points were limited to the upper extremities and the left leg. More recently chest leads were added and, occasionally, an electrode may be placed in the esophagus for special studies in which the back portion of the heart must be examined. The right leg is used in some machines as a ground.

To obtain a correct tracing, it is recommended that the patient avoid smoking for about one hour before the recording, as well as a heavy meal or cold drinks. Whenever possible the patient should be supine, since sitting may alter the position of the heart and thus change the electrical pattern.

As the impulse spreads over the heart from the atria to the ventricles, two types of waves are registered. They are the P wave, which is small, due to the spread over the atria, and the QRS wave, which is much larger and represents the spread through the ventricles. The phase of recovery of the ventricles is indicated by the T wave. The electrocardiogram can only show the electrical activity of the heart muscle, it cannot signalize whether or not the muscle is contracting well.

The electrocardiogram chiefly serves two purposes. First, it will indicate whether or not the excitation wave is proceeding normally or if interference, due to illness, forces the wave to spread abnormally.

Similarly, it will indicate the path and speed of the recovery wave. The second value of the electrocardiogram is the recording of arrhythmias, which mean a change in the normal rhythm of the heart. Fortunately, most of these arrhythmias are harmless, but occasionally can be caused by more serious conditions which require medical attention. The electrocardiogram can often show a differentiation between these two categories and thus can help not only to reassure the patient but to provide foundation for proper treatment.

Since each person's heart has its own characteristics, each electrocardiogram is specific. The only exception to this is found in identical twins. This specificity of the electrocardiogram is so definite that it has been suggested to use the electrocardiogram as a means of identification. However, this is not practical since changes may occur rapidly in the course of disease.

LIMITS OF THE CARDIOGRAM

Since innumerable variations are visible in normal electrocardiograms, the interpretation of the tracings requires long experience to differentiate normal variations from pathological conditions. Too often a patient is haunted for life by the statement that his electrocardiogram is abnormal, while actually he has only a rare variant of a normal tracing. Moreover, the finding of a normal electrocardiogram does not necessarily indicate a normal heart. Lesions in the heart muscle, situated in such a manner as not to disturb the spread of the excitation in the major part of the muscle, will not be recorded, and a normal tracing will be obtained.

Electrocardiography is only one of the many mechanisms at the disposal of the physician and should be used in conjunction with the other methods of examination such as auscultation, measurement of the blood pressure, X-ray examination, and others. Just as numerous findings may vary on repeated examinations, so may the electrocardiogram differ from one tracing to the next. The heart has such excellent recuperative power that complete normal function and findings are possible after recovery from an inflammation of the muscle, known as myocarditis, particularly after viral infections, such as poliomyelitis or mumps, or even after the patient has recovered from diphtheria.

CARDIOGRAM AND CORONARY SCLEROSIS

The contribution of the electrocardiogram to the diagnosis of coronary sclerosis is especially valuable. Changes often appear early and are the only significant indication in the course of a routine examination. In many instances even the person's medical record fails to reveal any symptom, and the diagnosis and recommendations are based solely on the electrocardiogram. Furthermore, serious arteriosclerosis of the coronary vessels may not be reflected in the electrocardiogram if the blood supply of the muscle is not impaired.

This was shown by studies made on the coronary arteries of young soldiers killed during the Korean War. Arteriosclerosis of these vessels was found in more than 70 per cent, and we know that in the age group over fifty the percentage is much higher. It can be concluded that the majority of our adult population suffers from this abnormality. However, coronary sclerosis becomes noticeable and the electrocardiogram becomes abnormal only when the narrowing of the blood vessels is sufficient as to impair the blood supply to the muscle, and in most instances this is not the case.

It is therefore evident that a normal electrocardiogram does not indicate the presence of coronary sclerosis as long as adequate blood supply is being maintained.

THE EXERCISE TEST

In many patients with disease of the coronary arteries, the blood flow which is ample at rest becomes insufficient during physical exertion when the heart requires more blood for the muscle. These patients may develop chest pain known as angina pectoris during this exertion, while at the same time electrocardiographic changes may occur. This observation prompted me many years ago, in 1933, to utilize the exercise test as a diagnostic aid. After thorough examination of the patient, an electrocardiogram is taken at rest. If all the findings are normal, he is then made to exercise, the degree of effort being gauged on his physical condition and record. If pain develops during the test, the patient must stop at once. After the exercise an electrocardiogram is taken at stated intervals and the variations studied. Certain modifications of this test have been introduced, such as establishing standards based on sex, age, and weight, but the basic principle remains the same: whether or not the blood flow to the working heart is sufficient to keep the muscle well supplied.

MYOCARDIAL INFARCTION

As a coronary vessel becomes occluded, the area of the muscle supplied by that vessel will be altered and eventually die. The condition is known as myocardial infarction and the result necrosis. This area will be electrically changed and will thus alter the electrocardiogram.

These electrocardiographic abnormalities may appear quite early, almost coinciding with the onset of the pain, or in some patients may be seen only after several days. The electrocardiogram permits the diagnosis of heart attack in approximately 98 per cent of the cases. Only when the muscular area involved is small and does not contribute much to the electrocardiographic pattern must a diagnosis of myocardial infarction be made on the basis of other criteria. For this reason, it is advisable to rely also on clinical evaluation and laboratory tests, before definitely ruling out this diagnosis.

The return of an electrocardiogram to a normal pattern, or normalization, following such injury depends on many factors and may never be complete although the patient may not have any further symptoms referable to the heart. Prognosis depends much more on the evolution of the arteriosclerotic process than on the electrocardiogram.

TYPES OF ELECTROCARDIOGRAMS

Certain types of electrocardiograms are seen in some congenital lesions of the heart and may contribute to the diagnosis, although other methods such as radiography with special techniques or cardiac catheterization usually offer more information.

When changes in the chemical composition of the blood are present, particularly with variations in potassium and calcium, characteristic changes appear in the electrocardiogram, permitting a diagnosis even before laboratory confirmation. Treatment of such deviations at that time may be life-saving.

In some endocrine diseases the electrocardiogram may reflect these variations and point to a diagnosis unsuspected previously. Perceptible changes appear also in certain vitamin deficiencies.

In cases of blunt trauma to the chest wall or following certain lung conditions, such as pulmonary embolisms, the electrocardiogram may be the only test that will reflect some abnormality.

In cases of irregularities of the heartbeat, also known as cardiac arrhythmias, the electrocardiogram can be diagnostic at a glance. This in turn may indicate whether or not the condition is a harmless arrhythmia or the manifestation of the development of heart disease. In the course of anesthesia or during the administration of certain drugs, evidence of some of these arrhythmias permits early change in the therapeutic regime. Although in some cases, the finer mechanism of these arrhythmias has not been interpreted, little doubt appears as to the possibility of a diagnosis from the electrocardiographic tracing.

Chapter XI

Ballistocardiograph and Heart Catheterization

Isaac Starr, M.D.

CARDIAC ABNORMALITIES may be divided into those concerned with the heart's structure and those associated with its performance as a pump. Among the latter, the strength or weakness of the heart muscle is of prime significance. The electrocardiograph does not reveal anything pertaining to this; the pulse, relied upon since medieval medicine to give information on the point, is far from infallible. The ballistocardiograph aims to provide a simple method of detecting the strength or weakness of the heartbeat. It can be applied to anyone without the slightest danger or discomfort.

As ordinarily employed, the ballistocardiograph provides a record, called the ballistocardiogram, of the forces acting on the body as a result of cardiac contraction. Many persons, when standing on a spring scale to weigh themselves, may have noticed that the pointer moves in time to their hearts. This movement is recorded in the ballistocardiogram. The cause is clearly understood. When the heart contracts, blood is expelled from it in a headward direction. When you fire a gun it kicks you in the shoulder, and for the same reason, when the blood starts headward, the recoil pushes the body feetward. An instant later the onrushing blood strikes the arch of the aorta, and the curve of the pulmonary artery and its headward movement is in large part arrested. This change of direction of the blood provides an impact which drives the body headward. Therefore, the two chief movements recorded in the ballistocardiogram are footward and then headward, and these are repeated every time the heart beats. Everyone's body sways back and forth as his heart beats, but the movement is too small to be noticed.

This motion is easily magnified and recorded with modern electrical equipment.

The first ballistocardiogram, a crude affair, was recorded by J. W. Gordon in 1877. The modern era began about 1938, when the instrument received the name used today, and systematic studies on patients were begun. At present in the world's scientific literature, a paper on this subject is published, on the average, once every four days.

Great improvement in the ballistocardiograph has been made in recent years. In one type of study, the patient lies on a light table suspended from the ceiling, free to move. The light table follows the motion of the body lying on it, and a record of the acceleration of such a table gives the force ballistocardiogram. These beautiful ultralow-frequency instruments are delicate and the electrical equipment is elaborate.

In another type of examination, the subject lies on a light stiff table held steady by a strong spring. A record of the movement of this table gives the force ballistocardiogram. This high-frequency apparatus is stronger and more durable than the preceding one described and the electrical equipment is simpler. It is, however, difficult to avoid slight movement between the subject and the table, and this may somewhat distort the record.

The shin bar method of William Dock is much simpler and less expensive than the table methods, but it is also cruder. The patient lies on any rigid surface, such as the floor, and a light bar is placed across his shins. Because the patient's tissues are elastic, his body swings back and forth as the forces generated by the heartbeats push it to and fro and this movement is recorded.

The simplicity of the shin bar method commends it to many doctors, but the properties of the body tissues affect the record, which, as a result, is a distorted version of the true force ballistocardiogram. However, this simple method will demonstrate cases of severe heart muscle abnormality, which would be overlooked by doctors relying solely on the methods of the past.

Skill and experience are necessary for the proper taking and interpretation of ballistocardiograms, for any movement made by the patient produces forces that affect the record. With a little experience, these noncardiac effects are readily recognized.

In medical practice, the ballistocardiogram is used to estimate the heart's strength. When the heart beats strongly, the record is large, and if weakly, the record is small. To measure this with confidence, the physician must have a standard with which the magnitude of the patient's record can be compared. Records from the table methods are much more readily standardized than those secured by the shin bar method.

The ballistocardiogram also indicates the coordination of the cardiac contraction. The diseased heart may lose its ability to contract smoothly and as a unit, and consequently the ballistocardiogram is distorted.

The use of the ballistocardiogram in the clinic has led to many interesting discoveries. It demonstrates that, as a person grows older, the heart, like the peripheral muscles, becomes weaker. In the group of patients whom I have studied and followed for twenty years, those with small records either died or developed heart disease in numbers significantly larger than those with large records. In many cases of structural heart disease, such as those following rheumatic fever, the strength of the muscle is not affected for many years. Smoking, which does not have any demonstrable adverse effect on the hearts of young persons, has a temporary effect on the hearts of many older people apparently in good health, and on a still larger number of those with coronary heart disease. An attack of angina pectoris is accompanied by definite weakening and incoordination of the heart, which recovers as the attack passes. In some cases of cardiac infarction or coronary thrombosis, the strength of the heartbeat is affected little, if at all, but in others, unhappily, the heart is hard hit and recovery may not take place. Drugs commonly used in heart disease, such as digitalis and nitroglycerin, usually, but not in every case, cause great improvement in the ballistocardiogram.

The ballistocardiogram provides easy access to information relating to the strength or weakness of the heart muscle and the coordination of its contraction. This information may be used to determine the severity of heart disease, and the amount of improvement occurring either spontaneously or as the result of treatment. It will also aid in distinguishing between effective and ineffective therapeutic measures and in identifying factors, like smoking, which appear harmful to certain patients.

CARDIAC CATHETERIZATION

In catheterization of the right ventricle, the tip of a thin flexible tube, about a yard long, is inserted into a vein at the bend at the elbow. As the operator feeds the catheter into the arm, the tip passes up the veins of the arm and, following the course of the larger veins, turns a half-circle and enters the right side of the heart, into the pulmonary artery and finally into one of the lungs.

That such a maneuver could be made without great risk to the patient came as a surprise to the medical profession. Cardiac catheterization was first performed by a German, Dr. Werner Forssmann, who did it several times on himself without ill effect. However, Dr. André Cournand, an American of French birth, and Dr. Dickinson W. Richards, working in Bellevue Hospital, New York, perfected the procedure. As a result of their work, all three shared the Nobel Prize in medicine for 1956.

Cardiac catheterization is a minor operation. Local anesthesia is administered before opening the vein of the arm. With this preparation the passage of the catheter does not cause the patient pain or discomfort. Even in the early days of the procedure difficulty was rarely encountered. Occasionally the heart, irritated by the presence of the catheter within it, loses its ability to contract properly, and occasionally a clot, formed inside a vein or in the heart, as the result of some diseased condition, has been pushed loose by the tip of the catheter and, swept into the lungs by the blood, lodges there and obstructs the circulation. Increased technical skill and careful selection of patients for catheterization have greatly reduced the number of complications.

USES OF CARDIAC CATHETERIZATION

The beneficial information given by cardiac catheterization is of three kinds. First, the examiner may measure the pressure at the tip of the catheter by connecting suitable apparatus to its free end. By this means the pressure in the central veins, in the cardiac chambers, and in the pulmonary artery can be appraised. The pressure in the pulmonary artery is abnormally elevated in certain types of pulmonary disease, and especially when a narrowed mitral valve of the heart prevents the free outflow of blood from the lungs. Abnormal differences in pressure, as the catheter tip is slowly advanced through the heart, aid the technician or physician in identifying cardiac abnormalities such as narrowing of those valves through which the catheter passes.

Second, information can be gained by the study of blood samples drawn through the catheter. Normally the venous blood has little oxygen, but the blood in the left side of the heart contains much more. Therefore, if blood passes through an abnormal communication from the left to the right side of the heart, this will be detected by an increase in oxygen content of blood samples taken through a catheter placed first in the great veins, then in the heart, and finally in the pulmonary artery. Also, the oxygen content of mixed venous blood, obtained through a catheter, may be used in calculations of the amount of blood pumped by the heart.

Third, solutions can be injected down the catheter. When solutions opaque to X rays are thus injected, a series of roentgenograms taken rapidly, like an X-ray movie, will show the cardiac chambers beautifully outlined. Furthermore, the progress of the opaque solution can be followed through the right heart, into the pulmonary artery, back to the left heart, and into the aorta. Anatomical abnormalities of the heart and great vessels may be shown clearly by such a technique. Also, a solution of a harmless dye may be injected through a cardiac catheter. This mixes with the flowing blood, and blood samples taken from the arms or legs provide information about the amount and rapidity of the flow of the blood and sometimes may reveal the presence of abnormal openings between the cardiac chambers.

Cardiac catheterization finds its greatest usefulness in the diagnosis of abnormalities of the pulmonary circulation and anatomic abnormalities of the heart such as are found most frequently in congenital and rheumatic heart diseases. Since some of these can now be corrected surgically, cardiac catheterization often provides information of great significance to the patient.

Catheterization of the *left* ventricle has proved much more difficult and hazardous than that of the right, and this procedure is not widely used on this ventricle at present.

Chapter XII

Angina Pectoris

MYRON PRINZMETAL, M.D., *and* REXFORD KENNAMER, M.D.

THE TERM angina pectoris is a medical phrase that designates a specific pain. The diagnosis of angina pectoris indicates that the blood supply of the heart muscle is *temporarily* inadequate for the active muscle. It is not completely and permanently cut off.

When any active muscle fails to receive enough blood to keep pace with its needs, pain results, whether it is a muscle in the legs, the arms, or in the heart. If the muscle that is temporarily receiving inadequate blood is the heart muscle, then the resultant pain is known as angina pectoris. In contrast, should the blood supply to a portion of heart muscle be completely and permanently cut off or occluded, the muscle would die and the proper term here would be heart attack.

Angina pectoris is a symptom, just as headache is the diagnosis of a particular characteristic or subjective sensation. Headache does not reveal whether or not the underlying cause is a brain tumor, brain abscess, meningitis, or some other ailment. Nor does the phrase angina pectoris disclose why the heart muscle is not getting enough blood to meet its needs. However, in both instances a single cause is so predominantly common that the symptom diagnosis has become synonymous with the underlying disease.

Certainly 90 to 95 per cent of all headaches are due to tension, and the proper diagnosis would be "tension state manifest by headache." In angina pectoris the overwhelmingly common cause is arteriosclerosis, hardening of the coronary arteries, or the blood vessels of the heart; the result of this hardening is that enough blood does not get through to the heart muscle. Therefore the proper diagnosis in these cases is arteriosclerotic heart disease manifest by angina pectoris. Nevertheless, we usually state simply that angina pectoris exists.

Infrequently the blood supply of the heart muscle is diminished because rheumatic fever has damaged the heart valves and adequate blood is prevented from getting out into the coronary arteries; or because of syphilis, which has damaged the openings of the coronary arteries; or by anemia when the total body supply may be so impaired that the heart muscle is inadequately nourished. The symptom diagnosis in these cases would also be angina pectoris but the underlying disease should be indicated.

Angina pectoris occurs as paroxysms, or attacks of short duration, although the underlying disease is present at all times. The actual attacks of angina pectoris are best explained as an imbalance in supply and demand of blood. The blood supply to the heart muscle may be completely adequate under the ordinary circumstances of daily life, but it can become insufficient if any increased demand is made upon it. This insufficiency is angina pectoris. The heart muscle is required to do some extra work and must have extra blood to accomplish this function. A demand is made by the heart muscle for an increased supply of blood which cannot be furnished because the "pipe lines," or coronary arteries, are usually afflicted with arteriosclerosis and cannot carry the extra load. Pain then results as the heart muscle cries out for more nourishment.

A person first becomes aware of angina pectoris when he is climbing a hill, playing tennis, having sexual intercourse, or is emotionally disturbed. In these efforts, the heart's work is increased and the heart muscle, in turn, demands an increased supply of blood.

Since the pain of angina pectoris is almost always in the chest, the phrase angina pectoris was derived from the Latin, signifying "pain in the chest." The term was first used in 1768 by Dr. William Heberden who gave a succinct description of the clinical symptoms:

> Those, who are afflicted with it, are seized, while they are walking, and more particularly when they walk soon after eating, with a painful and most disagreeable sensation in the breast, which seems as if it would take their life away, if it were to increase or continue: the moment they stand still, all this uneasiness vanishes.

It remained for the same physician who gave us smallpox vaccine, Edward Jenner, in 1778, to relate the clinical symptoms of chest pain to the underlying disorder in the coronary arteries. After the study of two autopsies, he observed:

> In the first of these I found no material disease of the heart, except that the coronary artery appeared thickened. As no notice had been taken of such a circumstance by anyone who had written of the subject, I concluded that we must seek for other causes as productive of the disease; but about three weeks ago . . . we found the same appearance of the coronary arteries as in the former case. But what I had taken to be an ossification of the vessel itself, Mr. P. discovered to be a kind of firm fleshy tube, formed within the vessel, with a considerable quantity of ossific matter deposited irregularly through it.

PAIN IN ANGINA PECTORIS

The pain in an attack of angina pectoris develops slowly, rather than with a sudden momentary onset. The pain increases gradually and becomes progressively worse until the exertion is diminished or stopped. With rest the pain gradually subsides and disappears in two to three minutes.

The pain is usually described as a pressure under the breastbone. However, it has been defined variously as a sensation of squeezing, heaviness, choking, fullness, aching, tightness, or burning. The pain is not restricted to the chest, but is ordinarily felt in the left arm and sometimes extends down to the left hand. In some instances, the pain radiates into the neck, or right shoulder, or right arm.

Occasionally, a person feels the pain in his jaws or gums, especially if the teeth are in a poor condition, and another feels the pain in the throat or tongue. Sometimes the pain passes right through the chest and into the back. Some persons do not have any chest pain, and notice the suffering only in the secondary areas such as the wrist, the arm, or throat. The pain in these parts of the body is usually characterized as aching or burning.

The severity of the pain is extremely variable from person to person, depending on his sensitivity. One individual may describe the pain as severe and intense and associated with great fear and sense of impending death. To another the sensation is so mild that he describes it as a discomfort rather than a pain. Some of these persons attribute the aches to heartburn or gas, and go for many months or years without seeking attention.

CAUSES OF ANGINA PECTORIS

Certain conditions exert secondary precipitating influences on angina pectoris. The two most common causes are food in the stomach and exposure to cold. It is not at all rare for a person in the early stages of the disease to be aware of the pain only when he exerts himself after a meal or in cold weather. The situation most favorable for the precipitation of angina pectoris is for a fat man to walk up a hill on a cold day after a heavy meal. Anemia and an overactive thyroid also serve as secondary precipitating factors.

Thus far we have been discussing the angina pectoris that occurs when an imbalance in the supply and demand of blood exists because of an increased demand for blood. However, angina pectoris occurs also when the fault is in the lack of blood rather than in the demand from the muscle. In such instances the relationship of pain to exertion may not be present. For example, the heart may be failing as a pump and as a result does not circulate enough blood through the coronary arteries to the heart muscle. In these cases the heart failure may have nothing to do with exertion and the anginal pain may occur even during the night, depending on the precipitating cause of the heart failure.

Recently, we studied a group of patients in whom the diminished blood supply appeared to result from a spasm of the diseased coronary arteries. This differing form of angina occurs usually while the patient is at rest, and some have found that it can be relieved by exercise. The pain is usually cyclic in character; that is, it comes and goes. Generally, it is more severe than exertional angina and lasts for longer periods of time. The attacks are frequently associated with disturbances in the rhythm of the heartbeat, giving rise to palpitation during the seizure. This newly observed type of angina produces an unusual electrocardiogram, quite different from that of the classical form of angina we have been discussing. Neither the pain nor the electrocardiogram can be reproduced by exercise. In fact, many of these patients can perform active, heavy work without precipitating the attacks of pain.

Few illnesses in medicine depend so much upon the history given by the patient for proper diagnosis. Intelligent, observant people are able to give the physician excellent descriptions of their pain as regards its location, severity, radiation, relationship to eating, smoking, and exercise, its duration, manner of onset and disappearance, relationship to emotional upsets, and other factors. Given proper data and observations, the physician can decide, without resort to laboratory tests, whether or not angina pectoris exists.

Whenever chest pain occurs, concern that the pain arose from the heart is immediately aroused. Many sources other than angina pectoris cause chest pain. Arthritis of the neck, painful muscles in the chest wall, hernias of the diaphragm, and esophageal spasms may be difficult even for the expert to differentiate from angina pectoris. The precordial aching described by patients with anxiety and nervous tension must also be considered in the differential diagnosis.

THE ELECTROCARDIOGRAM

The electrocardiogram is the only diagnostic tool of any significance in establishing whether or not a person has angina pectoris. It has its limitations, however. If the electrocardiogram is taken during a spontaneous attack of angina pectoris or an induced attack, its value as a diagnostic tool is greatly enhanced. If during an episode of pain the electrocardiogram fails to show a certain deviation or pattern, it is doubtful that angina pectoris exists.

The reverse is also true. If an electrocardiographic pattern of angina pectoris can be induced by exercise, then the diagnosis is considered more likely. Such an electrocardiographic study is now usually made by the physician in his office and is known as an EKG exercise test. The patient walks up and down two steps following which the electrocardiogram is taken. The test is frequently known as Master's Two-step Test, after the doctor who has done most to popularize and standardize it. False positive and false negative results do occur, however, in this test. Therefore, the electrocardiogram can only be considered as an accessory tool in making the diagnosis of angina pectoris.

Certain people are more prone to develop angina pectoris than others. The predisposing causes are the same as those which provoke arteriosclerosis. Men are more likely to have the disease than women who have not gone through the menopause, and high blood pressure and diabetes increase the likelihood of angina pectoris. Hypercholesterolemia, a condition of too much cholesterol in the blood, also increases the tendency to this symptom. Disorders of the thyroid gland will often precipitate episodes of this pain. Therefore, when a person is suspected of having angina pectoris, studies in addition to an electrocardiogram are likely to be made by the physician.

OUTLOOK IN ANGINA PECTORIS

The person who has developed a serious disorder is anxious to know what the course of his illness will be and what complications he may expect. What treatments are available and what can be done to prevent any complication?

The most common course of angina pectoris is for the attacks to continue over a period of years. Usually a gradual increase in the frequency of the attacks occurs, and they are stimulated less and less by exertion or excitement. Occasionally a patient may have attacks for a month or more, and then may be free of the pain for as long as a year. Sometimes new blood vessels develop and take over the function of the diseased ones, and the patient becomes permanently free of the pain.

In the course of the disease approximately one-half of all angina pectoris patients will develop a heart attack. This is the most serious complication of the ailment. In some patients the heart attack serves as a paradoxical form of cure for the angina pectoris, in that they become free of the seizures of anginal pain after the attack. In our experience this phenomenon is more likely to be seen in those patients who had the variant type of angina which occurs primarily at rest.

TREATMENT OF ANGINA PECTORIS

The treatment of angina pectoris can best be understood by considering three aspects of the therapy: 1) what to do for an attack; 2) what to do to prevent attacks; and 3) what to do to prevent a complication.

When an attack of angina occurs, the person should cease all activity. If he is walking, he should stand still immediately. In the vast majority of instances this procedure alone will usually relieve the pain in one or two minutes.

The drug used to ease an attack of pain is nitroglycerin. This small pill is placed under the tongue where it is absorbed. In practically all cases of true angina pectoris, nitroglycerin will bring about relief of the pain in approximately one minute. Every person with angina pectoris should carry nitroglycerin and use it for any attack which has not been relieved within one minute of ceasing activity. This drug may have some undesirable effect such as flushing or throbbing in the head, but these effects are usually overcome by adjustment of the dosage. Nitroglycerin is a remarkably effective drug, remains so despite repeated use, and is never detrimental to the patient.

Some persons, and some physicians, prefer to use the nitrite in the form of amyl nitrite ampules, which are as effective as the nitroglycerin. On breaking the ampule, the patient inhales the vapor. Most people, however, find the nitroglycerin pills more pleasant, more convenient, and more economical.

PREVENTION OF ANGINA PECTORIS

The prevention of angina pectoris is less definite than the treatment of an attack. Those individuals who are observant seek to learn what tasks and activities they can perform without bringing on an attack. It is essential that they learn the level of activity they can live within without precipitating an attack. Nitroglycerin can be used prophylactically to prevent seizure. If the person discovers that walking to the mailbox each morning hastens an attack, he may find it wise to take a nitroglycerin before starting out and thus prevent the pains. Sedatives and tranquilizers are effective in preventing angina pectoris in highly emotional people.

Recently, a group of drugs commonly called psychic energizers have been found to be effective in preventing the pain of angina pectoris, but drugs of this type must be used with great precaution since they relieve the person of his warning sign without doing anything to improve the condition.

The ideal preventive drug would be a long-acting one that could be taken by mouth and would be effective as nitroglycerin is. Most critical observers agree that such a drug is not yet available.

In some instances the frequency and severity of the attacks of angina pectoris seem unbearable. Furthermore these patients may be using 50 to 100 nitroglycerin tablets a day, although they may be at almost complete rest, and life itself becomes gravely endangered. Surgical procedures have been devised to relieve such conditions. Some of these operations are essentially for the relief of pain while others have the theoretic objectives of improving the blood supply to the heart muscle. These procedures must still be considered in the formative stage and have not yet reached a work-a-day usage in the treatment of angina pectoris.

One helpful approach to therapy of angina pectoris has been to reduce the work of the heart by lowering the metabolism of the patient. This is accomplished by reducing the activity of the thyroid gland. The most successful method achieving this has been through the use of radioactive iodine. The iodine is picked up by the thyroid gland which is subsequently depressed by the radiation. Often a severe degree of hypothyroidism must be produced to prevent attacks, and many patients find the induced disease of hypothyroidism as unpleasant as the angina pectoris, especially since the treatment serves only to relieve pain and does nothing to improve the underlying disorder.

Since every person with angina pectoris is a likely candidate for a heart attack, consideration must be given to the prevention of this serious complication. In recent years, drugs have been increasingly used to thin the blood and thus prevent the occurrence of a blood clot in the diseased coronary artery. Evidence is accumulating that this may be of value. However, the procedure is complicated, time-consuming, and expensive. Therefore, this particular type of therapy has been confined primarily to those severe conditions that appear to be on the verge of a heart attack, as indicated by an excessive increase in the frequency and severity of attacks of angina.

HYGIENE OF ANGINA PECTORIS

Certain rules of general health are as applicable to the patients with angina pectoris as they are to a patient with arthritis, tuberculosis, or diabetes. Too many people are pseudomedical authorities and become so involved in the intricacies of therapy that they overlook the significance of everyday factors. The role of diet, weight, exercise, smoking habits, drinking habits, home life, tension, frustrations of work—and avoidance of unproven therapies—cannot be overemphasized to the person with angina pectoris.

What about diet and weight? An overweight person with angina pectoris should reduce until he is at ideal body weight. Weight loss can only be brought about by a diet that is low in calories. In the light of modern knowledge, it is advisable to lower the caloric intake by eating a diet that is also low in saturated fats.

What about exercise? Patients with angina pectoris should definitely exercise. Walking is an excellent form of physical activity for these people. They should find by trial and error their particular tolerance as regards distance and speed of walking. Most patients find that they are gradually able to improve their tolerance.

What about smoking? Ideally, patients with angina pectoris should stop smoking. Occasionally this will bring about a dramatic reduction in the frequency of the attacks.

What about sex? Sexual indulgence is permissible, even if the person must take a nitroglycerin in order to avoid pain during the act. Frank discussion should be encouraged with the partners in order to avoid depression and marital discord.

What about hormones? The use of hormones is not indicated in the treatment of angina pectoris, except for experimental purposes. Much has been said recently about the use of female hormones in coronary artery disease, but at present these drugs do not occupy an impressive place in the treatment of angina pectoris.

What about alcohol? Patients with angina pectoris may use alcohol in moderation. Liquor does not have any specific value, but the tranquilizing effect and sense of well-being that accompany moderate drinking may be beneficial to many people. However, the caloric value of cocktails must be considered by those persons who are trying to lose weight. Also, it is imperative to remember that the patient must not come under the influence of alcohol to the extent that he overeats or performs excessively any other activities.

SUMMARY

Angina pectoris is the pain that results when heart muscle temporarily fails to receive an adequate blood supply. The underlying cause is usually hardening of the blood vessels of the heart. The common precipitation sources are physical exertion or emotional upsets. The acute attacks are best relieved by nitroglycerin tablets. Characteristics of the pain, complications, prognosis and therapy have been discussed.

CHAPTER XIII

High and Low Blood Pressure

ARTHUR M. MASTER, M.D., *and* RICHARD P. LASSER, M.D.

BLOOD PRESSURE is the pressure which is maintained in the aorta and in the major arteries of the body by the forceful pumping action of the heart or, more specifically, by the left ventricle, which is the major working part of the whole cardiovascular system. The left ventricle is a powerful muscular sphere. It contracts rhythmically, forcing blood with each heartbeat into the aorta and its branches, which then conduct the blood to every cell in the body to bring oxygen and nourishment, to remove wastes, and to control the body temperature. These are the major functions of blood circulation. The blood then returns to the heart through the *veins* after having given up its oxygen, is passed through the lungs by the pumping of the right ventricle, reoxygenated, and returned to the left ventricle to repeat the cycle. Thus, the system may be compared to the cooling apparatus in an automobile, in which the water pump (heart) forces water (blood) past the moving parts to remove heat, hence to the radiator to cool the water, and back to the pump to repeat the cycle. The water must be kept under pressure to keep it moving rapidly. Similar considerations are involved in the circulatory system, where it is also necessary to maintain a pressure so that the blood will move rapidly through the circuit.

The pressure within the arteries is not a steady flow, as in a river, but has waves, as in an ocean. The wave is created by the contraction of the left ventricle which flings blood into the aorta, raising the pressure to its highest level. This occupies slightly more than one-third of the time of each heartbeat. During the remaining two-thirds, the heart rests and refills with blood, and the pressure in the aorta and in the other arteries recedes and falls to the lowest level just before the next contraction begins. The highest pressure is called the systolic pressure; the lowest is called the diastolic pressure.

By international agreement, these pressures are expressed in terms of millimeters of mercury, that is, the height to which a vertical column of mercury would be lifted by the pressure in the arteries. It could be expressed in terms of pounds per square inch, with which we in America are more familiar; however, the millimeter scale is more widely used throughout the world. The numbers written down by the physician represent the height of the mercury column regardless of whether or not the instrument used is a true mercury manometer or the small, round gauge type. Thus, when the physician says that the systolic pressure is 140, he means that it is of sufficient force to raise the mercury column 140 millimeters above the zero level. Since pressures are always measured in the same unit, it is not necessary to specify millimeters of mercury each time. The symbol for millimeters of mercury is mm.

Historically, the cardiac cycle—the movement of the blood around the body—was not recognized until it was demonstrated by William Harvey in 1628. The belief then was that the arteries were filled with air and that the pulse represented the transmission of air through the lungs into the arteries. The first actual measurement of blood pressure was made in 1733 by Stephen Hales who determined the blood pressure of a horse by inserting a glass tube into an artery of the leg and then measured the height to which the column of blood rose. In the same way, he measured the blood pressure of sheep, dogs, and other animals, and achieved results that were remarkably correct. Later direct measurements of blood pressure were similarly made in man. Obviously, this was not practical, and many instruments were devised to measure pressure indirectly. The modern instrument was developed by an Italian, Scipione Riva-Rocci, at the University of Padua in 1896. It consists of two parts, an inflatable rubber cuff or band, which is placed about the upper arm, and a mercury manometer. As the cuff is inflated, the pressure compresses the arm and gradually squeezes shut the large arteries of the arm. The amount of pressure in the cuff necessary to accomplish this is a measure of the systolic or maximum blood pressure in the arteries. This point is determined by observing the disappearance of the pulse beat at the wrist or the disappearance of sound when a stethoscope is applied over the arteries at the elbow. The technique with the stethoscope now universally used was described by a Russian physician, Nikolai Korotkov, in 1905. With the stethoscope, the diastolic pressure may also be ascertained. Occasional errors may occur, particularly with children, when the size of the cuff must be reduced and, conversely, with persons who have large arms where the blood pressure may be overestimated. In fact, in some obese persons a true reading of the blood pressure is almost impossible.

Blood pressure is determined not only by the power of the heart and the quantity of blood expelled but also by another significant factor, which is the resistance to the flow encountered chiefly in the smaller vessels called the arterioles. These arterioles have a strong muscular coat and can change their diameter rapidly, thereby either offering increased resistance to the flow by closing down or decreased resistance to the flow by opening up. These little vessels are the site of the entire problem of high blood pressure, for according to their behavior the level of pressure is in large measure determined. If they perversely obstruct blood flow, the heart must beat harder and raise the pressure higher in order to force the blood flow past this obstruction. This is the situation in hypertension, and it is the reason that the heart is affected and fatigued in the person with high blood pressure. If the arterioles dilate too greatly, pressure fails. Considering that blood pressure is determined by the interplay of many separate factors, the body must coordinate and regulate these to maintain a stable pressure.

The level of blood pressure is maintained by a whole series of self-regulating or feed-back mechanisms within the aorta and the arteries to the brain. These mechanisms are designed to keep the blood pressure at a stable level. If the blood pressure for any reason decreases, they will stimulate the heart to beat faster and stronger and cause the arterioles to increase their resistance, so that the pressure will rise back to its previous level. These mechanisms function every time a person stands. They also operate during hemorrhage. Conversely, if the pressure rises higher than normal, these reflexes automatically slow the heart and dilate the arterioles to reduce the pressure. All this occurs totally automatically and unconsciously.

In addition to these unconscious, self-corrective controls, the blood pressure is also most responsive to stimulation by the conscious nervous system and can be affected by fear, joy, pain, temperature, and, in short, the entire gamut of human emotion. Ordinarily, unpleasant experiences, such as those associated with cold, pain, fright, and tension, cause a rise in blood pressure. Pleasant experiences, like warmth, sleep, and relaxation, lower the blood pressure. These are a few of the obvious forces which stimulate the conscious system, but each person has subconscious forces that represent pain or fear or anxiety whose cumulative effects over long periods of time may cause permanent elevation of blood pressure. Increased weight, particularly obesity, will elevate the blood pressure. Noticeable loss of weight from any cause, from a disease such as tuberculosis or excessive dieting, will usually result in low blood pressure. Furthermore, hereditary, racial, and environmental factors may be involved. Some families have a tendency to pressures on the low side and other families unfortunately have a strong tendency to high pressures, even at young ages. Oriental and Indian people seem to have a consistently lower blood pressure than Europeans or Americans. The presence of an environmental factor is shown by studies in which Chinese people living in this country were compared with Chinese people living in China. Those living here showed a consistently higher pressure than those living in China, possibly because of a slower pace of life in the older civilization. A small study was also made of Chinese who lived here for a time and then returned to China whereupon their blood pressure showed a tendency to return to lower levels.

Pressure also rises gradually with age and is somewhat different in the two sexes.

NORMAL BLOOD PRESSURE

Even after extensive experience, the concept of what constitutes a normal blood pressure is not yet entirely settled. Two schools of thought obtain. One believes that the highest level in the adult which can be considered normal is 150 systolic and 95 diastolic, regardless of age or sex. More recent studies, ours among others, indicate that this interpretation is too rigid, and that it would be wiser to consider the limits more extensively and establish them for each sex separately and in accordance with age. This opinion is supported by studies of the average pressures of large groups of healthy people.

The average normal blood pressure at birth is about 80/46. (The first number and highest always indicates the systolic; the second number, which is the lower, always designates the diastolic pressure.) The pressure then rises sharply during the first ten days of life to about 100/60, with a more gradual increase during the first month; then there is little change until seven to eight years. During adolescence, the pressure rises continuously, more steeply and more slowly during early adulthood. From twenty to twenty-four years the average normal pressure is 122/76 in men and 116/72 in women. A sex difference is already apparent. Men have slightly higher pressure than women in the early years of adult life. At thirty-five to thirty-nine years the pressure is 127/80 in men and 124/78 in women, and at fifty to fifty-four years the pressures are 134/83 and 137/84 respectively. Note that after the age of forty-five or fifty, the blood pressure in normal females is higher than in males. At seventy to seventy-five the average blood pressure in men is 146/81 and 159/85 in women. The blood pressure then remains constant in men to the end of life. In women after the age of seventy to seventy-four some gradual decrease is noted until, at the ultimate span of life, 110 to 115 years, it becomes equal to that of men.

This description pertains to the *average* normal person, but a considerable range of normal is permissible and therefore only a physician should interpret these values. A suggested standard is given in Table I, which should supplant such erroneous rules of thumb as 100 plus the age, or 120 plus one-third of the age, and others.

TABLE I

Average Normal Blood Pressure

(apparently healthy persons, 20 to 106 years of age)

Age Group	Males Systolic	Diastolic	Females Systolic	Diastolic
20–24	123	76	116	72
25–29	125	78	117	74
30–34	126	79	120	75
35–39	127	80	124	78
40–44	129	81	127	80
45–49	130	82	131	82
50–54	135	83	137	84
55–59	138	84	139	84
60–64	142	85	144	85
65–106	145	82	156	84

As pressure is easily elevated by emotion, the visit to the doctor may be sufficient to give a falsely high result in an emotional person. Therefore the physician tries to maintain an atmosphere of calm and to take the pressure repeatedly either during the same visit or after several visits in order to ascertain its true value. Often the pressure has been found to decrease 10 to 20 mm. in two successive readings only ten minutes apart. Nothing is accomplished by overemphasis on minor changes in blood pressure from visit to visit. The patient often pays entirely too much attention to this single aspect of the examination. Apparently, some persons with pronounced fluctuations in pressure may in the future develop permanently elevated pressures.

HIGH BLOOD PRESSURE, OR HYPERTENSION

Hypertension is one of the most serious diseases. Much progress has been made in the past ten years toward effective treatment and better understanding of the mechanism of hypertension. The basic cause of high blood pressure, however, is still elusive in the vast majority of cases. The disease is called essential hypertension for lack of a more specific terminology. Some difference of opinion prevails concerning how high the blood pressure must be before it is considered abnormal. A single level cannot be considered abnormal at all ages in both sexes because average normal blood pressure rises constantly with age until sixty-five years and is significantly higher in normal women after the age of forty-five. Therefore, we have constructed a table of abnormal pressure for each five-year age group and for each sex. Table II is a tentative guide for the physician and is not intended for interpretation by the patient. We include it only to give some ideas as to how the physician formulates his judgment.

TABLE II

High Blood Pressure*

Age Group	Males Systolic	Diastolic	Females Systolic	Diastolic
20–24	150	96	140	91
25–29	150	96	140	92
30–34	153	98	148	97
35–39	155	101	152	98
40–44	159	100	161	101
45–49	164	104	170	105
50–54	173	106	180	109
55–59	176	107	182	108
60–64	184	110	189	111
65–106	190	102	212	113

* This is intended only as a simple guide to abnormal pressures and should be interpreted only by the family physician.

The measurement of blood pressure is only one aspect of the entire medical examination and must be evaluated for each patient separately. In general, studies by insurance companies have shown that persons with the abnormally high pressures described in Table II have a much higher rate of heart attacks, heart failure, kidney and vascular disease. A significant decrease is also noted in their life span and individual variation is great. Thus, some people endure moderate or even severe elevations of blood pressure extremely well while others do not. Particularly is this true of women, many of whom with extremely high blood pressure for twenty and thirty years seem to have perfect health. We do not know why women seem to tolerate high pressures better than men. Furthermore, elevation of the *diastolic* pressure is much more serious than elevation of the systolic pressure. A constantly high systolic and diastolic pressure, even after rest, is more drastic than a fluctuating one.

The figures in our table represent high blood pressure of a considerable degree; nevertheless, persons with permanent lower values may also suffer the consequences of hypertension because of differences in physical constitution.

Although most cases of high blood pressure are without a known source, some specific causes have been recognized. The physician will usually conduct a diagnostic survey to make sure that such causes do not exist before calling the disease essential hypertension. Diseases of the kidney, such as chronic infection or nephritis, are predominantly associated with high blood pressure. The role of the kidneys in elevating blood pressure has been intriguing for many years. For some time physicians have known that persons with kidney disease showed evidence of high blood pressure, but the relationship was not clearly manifest until an ingenious experiment performed by Dr. Harry Goldblatt. He placed a clamp about the arteries that carry the blood to the kidney, but instead of closing it off entirely, he merely tightened it so that the blood supply to the kidney was reduced but was not so small as to cause the death of the organ. In these circumstances, he observed the development of high blood pressure in dogs. Further studies showed that the kidney with inadequate blood flow produced certain hormonal substances which were secreted into the blood stream and which were capable of elevating blood pressure. For a time this appeared to be the solution to the entire problem. Unfortunately, studies of humans demonstrated that in the vast majority of cases, occasional kidney disease was not the cause of essential hypertension. Sometimes, however, a clot in one of the arteries to a kidney can produce the definite obstruction and may produce high blood pressure, in which case removal of the diseased kidney may reduce the blood pressure to normal. Similarly, congenital (inborn) defects of one kidney, or infection of one kidney, may produce high blood pressure and if the involved organ is removed, the blood pressure falls. X rays of the kidney may reveal such a condition.

Among other remediable causes of hypertension which should be sought for in all children, adolescents, or young adults with high blood pressure is a congenital constriction of the aorta, called coarctation of the aorta. This condition produces the interesting phenomenon of a high blood pressure in the arm and a low one in the legs. Such constriction of the aorta can be successfully treated by an operation in which the constricted portion is removed and the aorta is restored to normal size.

Some glandular conditions, such as overactive thyroid, may also result in high blood pressure, in which case the systolic blood pressure is usually elevated and the diastolic blood pressure normal. Heart rate is also increased and other characteristic signs are apparent.

Another rare cause of hypertension is a tumor of the adrenal glands. The hypertension is usually of a fluctuating type, normal at times and exceedingly high at others. These glands secrete a substance called adrenalin which has the capacity of raising the blood pressure rapidly. In bending over, a tumor of this type may be squeezed and caused to secrete large amounts of adrenalin all at once. As a consequence, blood pressure suddenly rises, the heart begins to pound, and the patient trembles and perspires profusely. Removal of the tumor completely cures the high blood pressure. Simple and effective tests are available which a physician can make in the office to determine whether or not such a condition exists. Although tumor of the adrenal glands is extremely rare, physicians are cognizant of it when they observe that severe high blood pressure occurs in attacks or even continuously.

Blood pressure in some women may become extremely elevated during pregnancy. This condition is called toxemia of pregnancy, and may be associated with retention of fluids, swelling of the legs, puffiness of the face, severe headaches and, in a high percentage of instances, with the loss of the infant. The true cause of this serious toxemia is not known, but limitation of salt intake and administration of drugs which effectively remove the salt from the body lower the blood pressure and give the mother a good chance for a normal infant. Women who experience such rises in blood pressure during pregnancy often develop permanent high blood pressure later.

In rare cases, lead poisoning is associated with an elevation of blood pressure.

Aside from these few specific causes which are uncommon, elevated blood pressure occurs mostly in persons who do not have any underlying disease. Possibly the arterioles of persons with high blood pressure react more violently than ordinary to normal circulating substances such as adrenalin and other kidney substances, and perhaps this causes permanent elevation of the blood pressure. Persons who develop essential hypertension are emotional, but generally of the type who suppress emotional expression. They are tense and sensitive and react with excessive suppressed rage and anxiety to most occasions, large and small. They tend to repress their conflicts. Possibly these inner tensions establish constant impulses which go to the brain, then to the nervous system and affect the small arterioles and cause them to tighten. If this continues day after day, the sensitivity of these vessels may be increased so that they maintain thickening and the increased resistance, thus causing permanent elevation of the blood pressure.

How this works, for example, may be shown in the operation of a lie detector. This machine is simply a sensitive, continuous measurement of respiration, pulse, and blood pressure. When the person is asked questions which do not cause conflict, nothing happens to these vital functions. However, when a question is asked which touches a sore point, and a lie is told, the body reacts by a slight elevation of blood pressure, a slight secretion of adrenalin, and a slight increase in the respiration and pulse rate. These reactions indicate that some slight conflict has been engendered and suppressed within the body. Probably, the continuous succession of such small shocks of fear, anxiety or pain, whether physical or emotional, may be effective in producing chronic elevation of the pressure. Obviously great numbers of persons subject to the same stresses and strains do not develop elevation of blood pressure. Nevertheless, these stresses cause reactions in those who are susceptible.

Persons with a family history of high blood pressure have a greater tendency to develop high blood pressure than those without such a family history. Whether or not this is a matter of personality development or true hereditary susceptibility of the blood vessels is unknown.

Overweight and obesity definitely tend to increase the blood pressure and favor the development of severe hypertension. Furthermore, these elevated blood pressures decrease to normal when the weight adjusts to normal. Weight reduction therefore is such a significant aspect of the treatment and prevention of high blood pressure. Overweight also increases the amount of work the heart must perform and obese individuals are usually subject to a shortened life span due to other illnesses, such as hardening of the arteries or gall bladder disease.

Salt or sodium chloride, particularly the sodium, may be one of the dangerous components of high blood pressure. In persons with essential hypertension sodium accumulates in the arteries and may be the cause of the abnormal reaction. If these people observe a diet with a high salt content, the blood pressure will rise even higher; on a low salt diet it often falls to normal levels. This is the basis of modern treatment, since we now possess effective drugs capable of removing salt from the body and of inducing a lowering of high blood pressure. Normal persons do not experience any change in blood pressure either with these drugs or with the consumption of large amounts of salt. Thus, at present, restriction or abstinence from salt is believed to be useful only for treatment and not as a preventive measure.

The adrenal gland also plays an important role in regulating salt within the body. It secretes a substance called aldosterone, which influences retention of sodium in the body. People with high blood pressure often excrete large quantities of sodium. Research is now progressing to develop drugs to counteract its effect and possibly in the near future, another means of controlling hypertension will be found.

In the past, a variety of other factors have been suggested as causes of high blood pressure: tonsils, abscessed teeth, gall bladder infection, and constipation. None of these conditions has been found to cause high blood pressure and their correction rarely, if ever, affects the disease. These ailments are, therefore, treated the same in people with hypertension as in those without.

Excess smoking does not seem to have any effect upon the blood pressure, except in certain susceptible persons whose hands become cold and sweaty after a few puffs of a cigarette. This reaction is an evidence of excessive stimulation of the sympathetic nervous system by the nicotine. In a small number of these, hypertension seems to be either provoked or maintained by smoking. Complete cessation of smoking will lower the blood pressure to normal.

Because of the caffeine content in coffee, excess coffee drinking may sometimes temporarily elevate blood pressure. Although coffee is not a cause of hypertension, it is probably advisable for those with high blood pressure not to drink it excessively.

Alcohol is not a factor in provoking high blood pressure. Nevertheless, those with severe hypertension must be cautioned, since alcohol taken in large quantities dilates the blood vessels of the brain and may render a person who has high blood pressure susceptible to a stroke. Alcohol in excess should therefore be avoided. However, we repeat emphatically that the advice of the personal physician should be sought and followed in all these conditions.

SYMPTOMS

A popular misconception is that elevation of blood pressure itself will cause all sorts of symptoms. Thus, a patient may say, "My blood pressure is up today; I have a tightening of the scalp." He may complain of a headache, a pain in the back of the neck, excessive fatigue, noises in the ear, or dizziness when, as a matter of fact, none of these symptoms is in any way due to the elevation of blood pressure. These discomforts are more often the result of other diseases or of a neurotic fixation upon psychogenic symptoms. This has often been demonstrated when people who do not have such symptoms prove, upon examination, to have exceedingly high blood pressures. Acute elevation of blood pressure is occasionally associated with severe headache, which is particularly pronounced on awakening in the morning. Immediate treatment may be required to lower such pressure.

High blood pressure exerts deleterious effects upon the heart, kidneys, brain, and blood vessels. The heart muscle under such circumstances must pump harder than normally and thus enlarges, much as the muscle of a weight lifter, as can be observed in the electrocardiogram and X-ray picture. This excessive strain produces eventual weakening of the heart, and the symptoms are shortness of breath on effort, shortness of breath when lying down, and swelling of the ankles or accumulation of excess fluid within the system.

Such congestive heart failure can be effectively treated. Occasionally, these attacks of shortness of breath masquerade as asthma. The enlarged and overworked heart is subject to a higher incidence of angina pectoris and heart attacks than the normal heart. In fact, in women, heart attacks are not too frequent below the age of sixty unless high blood pressure or diabetes is also present.

In a small proportion of cases, the kidneys become diseased and are unable to eliminate the wastes from the body, and a condition called uremia develops. Uremia is always serious, but can be controlled with prompt, proper treatment.

Probably the most feared consequences of high pressure is a stroke. A stroke may be due either to a rupture of the blood vessels or to the formation of a clot in an artery within the brain. The person who has had a stroke lapses into coma and upon return to consciousness reveals paralysis of one or more parts of the body, as of an arm or a leg. Milder cases may occur, with only minimal changes such as weakness of an arm, temporary loss of strength of a leg, impairment of speech, or a change in personality and judgment. These paralyses and weaknesses usually are not completely permanent, and gradual improvement in function ordinarily occurs. Remarkable rehabilitation has been accomplished with modern physiotherapy.

A stroke is due to a clot within a large artery, and may sometimes be treated by the administration of anticoagulants, substances which keep the blood from clotting. For the prevention of strokes, the blood pressure should be controlled gradually in those who have extremely high pressure. Severe emotional upsets, family quarrels, and excessive alcoholic intake should be particularly avoided.

To give a complete picture of high blood pressure in this discussion, some of the serious consequences which may occur have been included. Persons with such complications should not become alarmed but should make a realistic adjustment to the disease, keep usefully employed, try to avoid excess tension, and visit the doctor periodically. We wish also to re-emphasize the enormous individual variability. Many people live long lives, even to old age, with high blood pressure, while others do not do so well even with modest elevation of blood pressure. The physician can determine the important factors and devise treatment accordingly.

TREATMENT OF HIGH BLOOD PRESSURE

About twenty-five years ago, little effective medication was available. Then doctors thought it advisable not to tell the patient about a moderate elevation of blood pressure for fear of inducing emotional strain and occasionally invalidism. This opinion is now somewhat revised. We know that abnormal elevation of blood pressure may shorten the life span and increase the risk of heart attacks, but we have extremely effective measures for lowering the blood pressure, with minimal side effects. The next step will be a true knowledge of the intimate cause of high blood pressure and, once we learn this, the disease will come under control.

The physician determines treatment by ascertaining whether or not the person has a permanent high blood pressure or simply a fluctuating pressure, high at some times and normal at others. (Tables I and II furnish a standard for each five-year age group and for each sex.) The physician then investigates to determine if a specific causative disease, such as an infected kidney, can be found and eliminated. Treatment of an overactive thyroid or occasionally the removal of an adrenal tumor may be indicated. If none of these diseases is found, as occurs in more than 90 per cent of cases, the patient is considered to be suffering from essential hypertension. Urinalysis, blood studies, electrocardiogram, and chest X ray may then be advised to determine the condition of the kidneys, heart, lungs, and other organs. The physician may also examine the retina or back of the eyes, through which he gains significant clues as to the severity of the disease and the state of the small blood vessels. On the basis of all these observations, he decides how serious the hypertension is and the course of its management.

For the great majority of cases, the physician will give reassurance that imminent changes will not occur, that the blood pressure can be readily controlled, that the elevation is not too serious, and that it is compatible with a long, useful, and natural life. Weight reduction may be advised, more frequent vacations, and possibly an adjustment to a more moderate pace of living. An ocean cruise for the tired executive or a slight revision of his goals and excessive ambitions may be helpful. Occasional sedatives or tranquilizers may be all that is necessary for the person who has temporary elevation of the blood pressure due to emotional instability. Minor variations of 5 or 10 points up or down should be disregarded and the blood pressure should not be watched like the stock market. The habit of taking frequent blood pressures should be discouraged, except in those few cases in which it is an essential consideration. People with ordinary degrees of hypertension should be encouraged to continue working and should not consider themselves as invalids, for activity is beneficial and they perform their work well. Work discourages concern with one's physical condition.

For hypertension of mild degree, the physician may employ the derivatives of the root of a plant grown in Egypt, whose effect has been recognized almost since the days of the ancient Pharaohs. Recent studies by Egyptian physicians showed that these properties have the capacity to lower high blood pressure. These drugs are marketed under various names such as Raudixin, Serpasil, Reserpine, Rauwiloid, and Singoser. These have proved to be extremely valuable sedative agents, since they have minimal side effects and can be taken safely over long periods of time. For cases of high blood pressure which do not respond satisfactorily, stronger products are available which act to block the effect on the autonomic nervous system. Known as ganglionic blockading drugs, they are marketed under such names as Ansolysen and Inversine. Research is making such progress that probably by the time this discussion is available, potent drugs will have been found. Therefore, the patient must be in touch with his physician to receive proper treatment. These drugs are used generally with patients in whom the high blood pressure is severe, in whom it is important to produce rapid, accurate, and considerable lowering of the blood pressure in order to spare the heart, brain, or kidneys. Proper management of drugs must be instituted with great precaution since they are associated with certain side effects which must be carefully controlled. The patient for whom such drugs are prescribed generally is required to see his physician frequently until a satisfactory treatment regime is established. In certain instances, some physicians have advocated that selected patients may be permitted to take their own blood pressure at home for self-regulation of these drugs. This has proved successful when the patient has been carefully selected and has been meticulously instructed by the physician who is interested in carrying out such a program. Constipation and difficulty with urination are side effects which can be regulated by the administration of other agents. Such drugs as Apresoline and Veratrum Viridae are also effective in lowering blood pressure. They may be used in the treatment of high blood pressure of persons with kidney disease.

Within the past two years, a significant leap forward has been taken in this field with the discovery that certain diuretic agents called chlorolhiazide (Diuril and Hydrodiuril), which remove excess salt and fluid from the body, have a pronounced action in lowering the blood pressure in persons with high blood pressure. The use of such diuretics in combination with the other medication previously mentioned results in a satisfactory lowering of the blood pressure with minimal side effects. Drug treatment should never be instituted or continued without a physician's advice and direction.

Historically, one of the first effective treatments was the institution of the rice diet, which was not, as most people thought, the eating of rice in addition to meals, but a diet consisting wholly of rice, rice products, and fruit. This diet proved to be extremely difficult to follow except under careful hospital management. There is no doubt that when a person followed such a diet meticulously, his blood pressure dropped remarkably toward normal. As was later shown, the chief benefits of his rice diet were attributable to its exceedingly low salt content. It has been almost entirely abandoned and replaced by modern drug therapy. However, in certain patients with severe high blood pressure and evidence of heart failure, who show tendency to the accumulation of salt and water in the body, it may still be necessary to resort to an extremely low salt diet. Such diets can now be made palatable.

Also, chiefly of historical interest is the surgical operation performed for relief of high blood pressure, wherein a portion of the sympathetic nervous system is removed. The operation is a major procedure considered only when severe hypertension is present that, in rare cases, fails to respond to medical therapy. Although the blood pressure in most operative patients falls satisfactorily immediately after the procedure, in a large proportion it returns substantially to the preoperative level within a year or two. Some patients, however, experience great relief for considerable periods of time. Moreover, a recent study showed that the operation has definitely prolonged life in a substantial number of patients.

LOW BLOOD PRESSURE OR HYPOTENSION

Probably the most common misconception about blood pressure is that low blood pressure is a disease. Actually, true low blood pressure or hypotension capable of causing symptoms is rare, and is usually a result of other diseases, such as tuberculosis, rheumatism, advanced cancer, and malnutrition, in which loss of weight is great. The pressure may be low in anemia, during hemorrhage from a bleeding ulcer, or following a heart attack when the heart beats too slowly because of disturbed rhythm (heart block). Some glandular conditions are associated with low blood pressure, such as underactivity of the thyroid (myxedema), of the pituitary gland (Symond's disease), and of the adrenal gland (Addison's disease). All these are specific disease entities, and low blood pressure is only one of the symptoms. Once the underlying disease is treated, the blood pressure rises. Drugs also may induce low blood pressure. Tranquilizers, aside from their sedative action, are mildly effective in lowering blood pressure. In certain susceptible persons this reaction may be greater, and they may have rather low blood pressure with resultant symptoms. This effect should be recognized and the drug discontinued. Occasional persons who have high blood pressure and are being treated actively to lower it may have a period of abnormally low blood pressure or hypotension which may require treatment.

Persons with disease of the nervous system are known to have a drop in blood pressure when they stand. This condition, called postural hypotension, occurs in older persons with diabetes and neuritis, sometimes in those with syphilis of the nervous system, and occasionally following strokes. Sometimes postural hypotension is found in otherwise normal people. It may be incapacitating and require treatment.

However, aside from these rather unusual instances, persons with relatively low blood pressure have definitely been shown by studies of insurance companies to live the longest and to have greater life expectancy even than people with average normal pressure. Thus, low blood pressure is an asset for the future and should be a source of satisfaction rather than one of worry.

Symptoms attributed to low blood pressure are fatigue, lack of stamina, poor concentration, constipation, dizziness, and middle-of-the-afternoon fatigue. These are largely psychogenic in origin. Those individuals who use as an excuse for all their complaints and anxieties a low blood pressure that is not the cause of their difficulties can often be greatly aided by psychotherapy. A slight raising of the blood pressure will not remove their psychologic abnormalities.

Fainting is an example of temporary lowering of the blood pressure. While commonly emotional, repeated fainting should be brought to the attention of the physician for thorough investigation, as it may occasionally be the result of one of the diseases of psychogenic origin.

Various definitions describe low blood pressure but not everyone agrees on how low is low. One definition is 100 mm. Hg systolic or less and a diastolic pressure of 60 mm. Hg or less, when standing in the upright position. We suggest that the dividing line be a little higher and consider values below 105/60 for men and 100/60 for women to be hypotensive.

Treatment is available for the occasional case of low blood pressure with true symptoms regardless of cause. These symptoms generally appear on standing erect or changing rapidly from a lying to a sitting position. The blood pressure falls because of the absence of proper reflexes to adjust to the upright position. Symptoms are due to inadequate amounts of blood being pumped to the brain. This results in temporary lack of oxygen, dizziness, blackout, and fainting may occur. Momentary loss of vision may also be noted, since the blood supply to the eye is temporarily inadequate. In these cases, drugs such as mephenterminesulfate (Wyamine or Aramine) may be given to raise pressure. They cause blood vessels to contract and stimulate the heart to pump forcefully. When pressure is seriously depressed, it can be raised by constant intravenous administration of a substance called Noradrenaline or Levophed. This procedure has saved many persons with severe heart attacks.

During operations prevention of low blood pressure in older people and in those with heart disease is important. The blood pressure may decline abruptly during anesthesia, particularly with spinal anesthesia, and the anesthetist must therefore administer the proper counteracting drugs to prevent this fall of pressure. Now that this danger has been recognized and can be avoided, operations can be performed on persons with heart disease without the risk which had previously existed.

While true low blood pressure does exist in persons who have certain diseases, low blood pressure in those who are not afflicted by such conditions is a blessing rather than a misfortune. Many psychogenic disorders have been attributed to low blood pressure, which do not disappear even if the blood pressure is raised. However, barring complications, this type of low blood pressure seems to lead to a longer life span.

CHAPTER XIV

Hardening of the Arteries:
Arteriosclerosis or Atherosclerosis

IRVINE H. PAGE, M.D.

HARDENING of the arteries, another name for arteriosclerosis or atherosclerosis, occurred in man at least 5,000 years ago. What is surprising is how little we know about it after all this time, especially since some 500,000 Americans will die as a result of it in 1960. Some investigators believe that this condition is on the increase, others insist that because people live longer, they have greater opportunity to develop this disease.

Investigations into the causes of arteriosclerosis were probably held back by the conclusions of many that it was not really a disease but merely a manifestation of old age and therefore inevitable. We now know that hardening of the arteries is not inevitable and that it usually begins and often may be extensive in youngsters.

Still another curious facet concerned in the history of knowledge of arteriosclerosis is the failure of astute physicans of a generation or more ago to recognize and treat what we now call a heart attack or "a coronary." Not until the early 1920s did Dr. James Herrick of Chicago convince the medical profession that such attacks are chiefly due to clots which originate in what are called the coronary vessels of the heart. These are the blood vessels that form a crown and sweep down over and within the heart muscle to supply it with blood.

This murky beginning of the study of so dangerous a disease has now been clarified. The past twenty years have seen a remarkable change in attitude by the public, physicians, and research workers. The public now knows that persons are not necessarily doomed when they have a heart attack caused by hardening of the arteries—President Eisenhower dramatized that. The physician knows that some reasonably good treatments are available for such heart attacks and that this is a disease and not just an accompaniment of old age. The research worker now knows that this is a fascinating field for work covering many areas of science, from organic chemistry to study of the Bantus in South Africa, the baboons in Central Africa, the animals in the Philadelphia zoo, or the Italians in south Boston. Hardening of the arteries, then, is a disease which most of us have and for some time will provide employment for many of us before its inner nature will be known so that it can be prevented and cured.

Arteriosclerosis is an important disease because it involves most of the arteries of the body at one time or another, notably those of the brain, heart, kidneys, and limbs. In each of these it causes characteristic manifestations. For example, in the brain it may lead to stroke or apoplexy, in the heart to coronary thrombosis, in the kidneys to a form of Bright's disease, and in the legs to gangrene or pain with even moderate walking, called intermittent claudication. Arteriosclerosis is the basis of all these serious bodily derangements.

It is not a "glamorous" disease, and develops slowly without overt symptoms in the beginning, but it is implacable and progressive. It does not make the headlines but it does the obituary columns.

THE NATURE OF THE DISEASE

Arteriosclerosis seems to differ somewhat from diseases caused by bacteria. In the latter, one organism or bacterium starts the process and if this is killed by an antibiotic, the disease usually abates. In arteriosclerosis, however, there does not seem to be any such single organism or cause. Rather, it is made of a constellation of facets, all of which contribute in some degree to the final manifest disease. In a way this explains why the public finds it difficult to understand what the scientists are talking about and why there seems to be such disagreement among them. The differences of opinion simply prove that hardening of the arteries is a young and vigorous field being tilled by young, vigorous, and usually inquisitive, questioning investigators.

The blood vessels actually do become hardened in a way, since they lose their elasticity, become thickened, and often calcium is deposited in them. More important, however, than the hardening is the thickening of the wall which encroaches on the lumen or canal of the artery. Little by little, less blood flows through it and the tissue being nourished by this blood begins to suffer.

A deeper look into this fascinating process reveals that substances of a fatty nature carried in the blood stream seem to get deposited within the blood vessel wall. Fat is the only substance needed in goodly amounts by the body which does not dissolve in water. The body then must maneuver to get this fat into solution and keep it there until it is transported to the tissues in the body where it will be burned for energy or stored to make some women cut the fine figures they do and make older men the sorry sag they so often sport. The trick that the body uses is to combine the fat with protein in the blood stream. The protein provides a vehicle for the transport of the fat. The only difficulty is that the combination is unstable and will break down to liberate the insoluble fat without too much provocation.

Blood in the blood vessels is under pressure (your "blood pressure"), and when it isn't, as one unsung investigator wrote in a fit of overconscientious anonymity, "Since this article was written, unfortunately one of us has died." This pressure tends to force the fluid of the blood through the blood vessel walls and this fluid carries with it the fat-protein combination. The blood vessel walls act much as a loosely-knit filter, letting most of the material through but holding back a small quantity. This small amount of material, particularly the fat-protein molecules just mentioned, probably causes arteriosclerosis. When this residue gets stuck in the vessel wall, it breaks down and frees the insoluble fat. This fat is irritating to the wall, and in an attempt to seal it off, scar tissue forms around it. Such are the beginnings of arteriosclerosis.

Another aspect of this condition is assuming more importance as we understand more about it. Recall that when you are cut, the bleeding is staunched by the formation of a clot made up essentially of a fine mesh consisting of strands of fibrin. Fibrin is a form of protein derived from the blood, which is formed much as industrial chemists produce polymers for synthetic fibers used in clothing. The body has ways of dissolving this fibrin as well as of forming it and normally the dissolving seems to keep up with the formation of these fibrin strands. In some people, however, more fibrin is deposited on the lining of the blood vessels than gets dissolved, and this may mean trouble. The cells that line the blood vessels grow over the fibrin strands and thus an elevated cushion or plaque is formed. The process is not normal, and usually fat is deposited in this thickened part of the vessel wall. This, then, is another way in which arteriosclerosis begins.

Hemorrhages can occur in these plaques and the resulting roughened surface can act as a nidus for the formation of a clot. When a clot or thrombus occurs in the coronary vessels, the heart muscle cries for blood, and a heart attack follows.

SOME CAUSATIVE FACETS OF ARTERIOSCLEROSIS

1) Heredity. Heredity plays a significant part in the production of arteriosclerosis. In some families, generation after generation, most of the members die before the age of thirty-five with coronary heart disease and elevated amounts of fat in their blood.

Formerly the view was generally accepted that nothing could be done about the hereditary aspect of disease. Today, since we are forewarned of what to expect, many of these developments can be averted. Even the old saw, "You should have chosen your parents more carefully," may some day make somewhat distorted sense because experimental evidence in animals indicates that sperm selection, radiation, and certain chemical treatments may alter the gene mechanism.

2) Hypertension. High blood pressure certainly accelerates the production of arteriosclerosis. This is not difficult to understand since the elevated pressure within the blood vessels tends to force more of the constituents of the blood out through the vessel wall. The chance is greater, therefore, of having more of it get stuck to start the mechanisms, already described, that result in arteriosclerosis.

Fortunately in the past fifteen years, treatment of hypertension has progressed from nothing to most effective procedures. Curiously this has been one of the unsung major victories of science. Economically, poliomyelitis is trivial compared to the millions of patients with hypertension. Rightly, the discovery of polio vaccine has been hailed as one of the major events of our century. However, so is the treatment of hypertension and the program developed for the prevention of rheumatic fever.

3) Exercise. The evidence that exercise retards the rate of production of arteriosclerosis is not strong but is appealing. Even in the absence of rigid scientific proof, it seems sensible and good hygiene to get regular and reasonably vigorous exercise. It is like taking a cocktail to dissolve the cholesterol in your arteries. It may not be true but it is fun.

4) Stress. Stress is certainly the most difficult factor of all to evaluate. To define stress for the individual is one of the first major hurdles and to keep the channel of thinking pertaining to it as objective as possible, not purely emotional, is a second considerable problem. I must candidly admit that many of my most respected investigator friends believe in it firmly. Stress to me seems to represent the challenge of life and without such challenge life would become relatively meaningless. Moreover, I do not know how to avoid stress, even if I would. Appealing to me is the belief of the possibility that stress affects the mechanisms which induce the formation of a clot and thus coronary thrombosis or apoplexy, rather than being directly involved in producing coronary or cerebral arteriosclerosis.

5) Sex. The sex factor is significant because the difference in the sexes not only represents a pleasant change in what might have been a dull homogeneous population, but it indicates a difference in death rate from arteriosclerosis of something like 3 to 1 with, of course, men representing the 3 and women the 1—a further example, as though we needed any, of the biological superiority of the female. Woman ceases to cut such a figure when she passes the menopause and then for all intents and purposes, or shall we say almost, she becomes like the male in her susceptibility to arteriosclerosis.

Modified female sex hormones are under study in attempts to incorporate within a tablet the part of femininity which protects against arteriosclerosis without the part that provokes attacks by males.

6) Diet. The most talked-about factor is diet. But then diet has al-

ways been talked about. The first aspect is the problem of obesity and the consumption of more calories than we need. I don't think anyone would defend obesity except a few of the obese. Obesity puts an extra load on the heart and on the pocketbook. It is indicative of too little load in the head and too much on the behind. Suggestive, but not conclusive evidence, associates obesity with a higher than usual incidence of arteriosclerosis.

Quite a different facet is the problem of whether or not the fat content of the diet determines the amount of arteriosclerosis. The answer seems to be that in some persons it does and that in others obesity plays a distinctly minor part. It is still uncertain whether or not the fat content of the diet of a nation truly reflects the incidence of arteriosclerotic heart disease. However, those countries with a high incidence of heart disease do in fact have a high rate of fat consumption. Whether or not the relationship is one of cause and effect is not known, though it is highly suggestive.

Furthermore, incontrovertible evidence is now available to demonstrate that the *kind* of fat in the diet helps to determine at least the level of cholesterol and fat in the blood, which may in turn help to determine the amount and kind of fat that may be deposited in the arteries. In brief, those fats of vegetable origin that are known as unsaturated fats seem to be the ones that depress, rather than elevate, the blood fats. On the contrary, the saturated animal fats tend to elevate them. Unsaturation simply is a measure of the avidity of fat to be oxidized in the air and thus ordinarily to become rancid. Most unsaturated fats are liquid at room temperature.

These facts about diet are stimulating and promoting the study of the practical application of food incorporating these fats. Corn oil, cotton seed oil, safflower oil, and soya oil all are under study. Once we have learned how to cook with these wholly successfully, it will remain to be shown that this factor is significant enough to reduce the death rate from coronary and cerebral disease of the blood vessels.

CONCLUSION

The next few years will doubtless see a rash of suggested preventives and treatments for arteriosclerosis. Although this disease is the commonest disease known to man, it has been largely overlooked. We may anticipate that before long, with the realization of its importance will come many bizarre views on its cause and cure. Food fadism will certainly be involved and this is one of the costliest bits of foolhardiness. Fortunately for the promoters and unfortunately for clarity in thinking, these fads usually are not dangerous unless carried to extremes. However, the taking of drugs to alter the rate of synthesis or destruction of fat and cholesterol could be potentially very dangerous. These should be tried only under the most carefully controlled experimental conditions. It is seldom wise to do something in the treatment of disease when you are not certain.

Work in the field of arteriosclerosis is progressing rapidly, building the solid foundation of knowledge necessary for ultimate solution of the many problems. It is fascinating and staggering to think how profoundly the prevention of arteriosclerosis would influence the people of the world. The solution will make the health of the people and their age far more important than their diseases.

In the meantime, certain common-sense rules are advisable which can be safely and, I think, effectively used in the prevention of arteriosclerosis. These are:

1) Understand heart disease and do not fear it.

2) Reduce weight if obese—eat less in the hope you will live longer to eat more.

3) If heredity is poor and blood cholesterol level is high, see your doctor and try to reduce the level by change in dietary habits.

4) Reduce blood pressure if it is elevated.

5) Reduce the proportion of solid animal fats to the liquid vegetable fats and reduce the total quantity of both. A balanced diet is important and extremes of all sorts should be avoided.

6) Increase the amount of regular exercise.

7) Avoid excesses of all kinds but don't miss anything.

8) Accept life's challenges, come to terms with the inevitable, and live as though you would live forever, and *in spirit you will.*

Chapter XV

The Child with a Deformed Heart

Willis J. Potts, M.D.

A few children are born with deformed hearts—we don't know why. If a mother has German measles during the first eight weeks of pregnancy, her baby is apt to have a deformed heart, defective eyes, and poor hearing. In the vast majority of children born with malformed hearts a definite cause for this calamity cannot be established. Actually, the percentage of children born with serious congenital heart disease is small, probably not more than one in three or four hundred.

The process of embryologic development of the heart, during the third to eighth week of pregnancy, is truly phenomenal, and so complicated that it is surprising not that defects do occur but that they are so rare. Approximately three weeks after conception when the fetus is less than a fourth of an inch long, the beginning of a heart appears as a bulge in a tiny blood vessel. The heart develops rapidly. It twists, bends, miraculously remolds itself to form compartments and valves, and begins to beat. By the time the fetus is eight to ten weeks old, the miniature heart is completely formed and has taken over its lifetime task.

Congenital heart disease is of special interest to those parents whose child is born with a crippled heart. Because a murmur is heard, or a chance X-ray picture is taken and shows enlargement of the heart, or symptoms such as pallor, failure to gain weight, too frequent colds, or cyanosis (blueness of the lips and fingers) present themselves, the child is sent to a heart specialist.

A rather wide variety of congenital heart defects appear in children; some are easily and permanently corrected, some can be improved, and a few are today hopelessly irremediable. It is most pleasant and satisfying to write about a heart defect that can be cured—the patent ductus arteriosus, the duct which connects the pulmonary artery with the aorta.

PATENT DUCTUS ARTERIOSUS

Before a baby is born, there is always a connection or ductus between the pulmonary artery, which carries blood to the lungs, and the aorta, which distributes blood to the entire body. Because the lungs of the unborn child are collapsed, full of water, and therefore resistant to blood flow, the tiny heart is unable to pump all the blood through them. The ductus arteriosus acts as an escape valve allowing the blood to be shunted into the aorta. At birth the lungs expand and immediately it becomes important that all the blood go through the lungs to supply the infant with oxygen.

The ductus arteriosus has fulfilled its function as an escape valve and ordinarily should promptly close. When it fails to do so, the blood flow through this opening is then in the opposite direction, that is, from the aorta to the pulmonary artery. If the ductus is wide, large amounts of blood escape from the aorta to the pulmonary artery and put a strain on the heart. Eventually the heart wears out because of excessive work.

The majority of children with an average-size ductus arteriosus, about one-fourth inch in diameter, appear perfectly healthy and can keep up with their playmates. If the ductus is large, heart failure may occur during the first year of life.

A diagnosis can usually be made by a physician with nothing but the aid of a stethoscope. A loud, rumbling, continuous murmur like the noise of a humming top is practically diagnostic of a patent ductus arteriosus.

In retrospect it seems strange that before 1938 nothing could be done for these children. In that year Dr. Robert Gross first successfully tied a string around a patent ductus and cured a child. Since then the surgical treatment of this condition has been perfected and is routinely successful. After the ductus has been surgically closed, the child has normal life expectancy. The most suitable age for operation is between two and five years, and it should be done before the heart begins to show signs of strain. If the ductus is large, heart failure may appear during the first few weeks of life and necessitate immediate operation. However, if the ductus is small, about three millimeters in diameter, the heart may not show any sign of strain before the age of thirty or forty.

COARCTATION OF THE AORTA

Some scientists perhaps with an admiration of big words concocted the term coarctation, which simply means constriction or narrowing. Why coarctation of the main blood vessel in the body should occur is still a mystery, and why it should practically always appear in the same place in the aorta, about six inches from its origin in the heart, is equally mystifying.

Children with coarctation of the aorta grow up quite normally and the condition is not suspected until a physician hears a mild heart murmur, takes the blood pressure, and feels for pulses in the legs. If the blood pressure in the arms is high, the pressure in the legs low, and the pulse in the groin weak or absent, the person has coarctation or narrowing of the aorta.

"What must be done about it?" parents want to know, and the physician explains that the most satisfactory time for operation has been found to be between the ages of seven and twelve years. To the question, "What will happen if nothing is done?", the answer is rather definite and clear-cut. The blood pressure in the arms, and more significantly in the head, will continue to rise and eventually, probably in ten to twenty years, a stroke will occur, the aorta may rupture, or the heart may go into failure. Operation is advised during late childhood, before irreversible changes have occurred in the blood vessels. Parents are apt to ask, "If the aorta is constricted, how does blood get to the lower two-thirds of the body?" This is a reasonable question. Nature is quite adaptable. Collateral vessels develop, which branch from the aorta above the constriction to the aorta below the constriction and carry enough blood to keep the lower two-thirds of the body properly supplied.

Rarely does a child with coarctation of the aorta have any attributable symptoms. In severe cases the child may complain of his legs being cold and "going to sleep." Although the blood supply to the major portion of the body is diminished, development is normal.

The operation is long and tedious but not particularly dangerous. The chest is opened and the constricted segment of the aorta is exposed. Special nonslipping clamps are applied and the narrowed segment is cut out. With carefully placed stitches the ends of the aorta are sewn together with fine silk. That is about all there is to the operation. It seems simple, nevertheless a certain amount of skill is required to sew the ends of so large a vessel together in such a manner that leaks will not occur. Resident surgeons in training get their experience in this particular yet tricky sewing on numerous dogs before they attempt to operate on a child.

BLUE BABIES

The typical "blue baby" is blue because the flow of blood to the lungs is partially impeded by an obstruction to the flow of blood through the pulmonary artery, and the baby doesn't get enough oxygen. Part of the blue blood returning from the body, unable to get to the lungs, escapes through a hole inside the heart and is pumped back through the body by way of the aorta. Obviously, the greater the obstruction to blood flow to the lungs, the more blue blood is shunted into the general circulation and the more serious is the child's condition. In mild cases the child's lips and finger tips are blue only after exertion; in severe conditions the child is constantly blue.

Many different kinds of congenital defects in the heart may cause blueness or cyanosis but the most common is the defect ordinarily spoken of as the tetralogy of Fallot.

Oxygen-starved infants with tetralogy of Fallot do not thrive; they gain weight slowly and because of constant discomfort are fussy and irritable. As they enter childhood they slowly learn to walk but have to stop frequently to "catch their breath," to get enough oxygen to proceed. The red blood-cell counts of such children, instead of being normal, between four and five million per cubic millimeter, are usually around seven million. This increase is nature's attempt to furnish more cells to carry oxygen to tissues. These children are such pitiable little creatures. Because they get blue when they cry and sometimes faint because of insufficient oxygen, parents naturally indulge them and they become quite spoiled.

Before 1945 nothing could be done to help these unfortunate children and many died during infancy or early childhood. All suffered because of varying degrees of cyanosis. In that year a miraculous thing happened. Dr. Alfred Blalock at Johns Hopkins Hospital in Baltimore had been doing experiments on dogs, trying to produce hardening of the pulmonary artery which ordinarily remains free from such changes. He reasoned that, since increased blood pressure causes arteriosclerosis or hardening in the aorta, if he connected a large branch of the aorta to the pulmonary artery, the increased pressure might produce hardening in a vessel not ordinarily so affected. Many operations were performed on dogs but the anticipated result was not obtained. One day a colleague, Dr. Helen Taussig, suggested that such an operation which increased the flow of blood to the lungs might be tried on children with tetralogy of Fallot who don't get enough blood to the lungs. Well, why not? The technique of connecting a branch of the aorta to the pulmonary artery was sharply improved. Parents were easily found who were willing to have this operation performed on their helpless and hopelessly sick children. The operations were magically successful. The medical world particularly, and the world generally, was electrified by the news of success, and parents everywhere grasped for the opportunity of having their oxygen-starved children relieved.

During the summer of 1946 Dr. Sidney Smith and I, by experiments on many dogs, perfected an operation described as aortic-pulmonary anastomosis, a method of shunting blood directly from the aorta to the pulmonary artery.

By means of the two methods of increasing blood flow to the lungs, thousands of children were given a new lease on life. The only fault inherent in both operations is that the deformities inside the heart remain uncorrected. True, more blood is sent to the lungs, but the heart is called upon to do extra work. Some children have done exceptionally well after these operations, while others have done poorly because of the excessive work load placed upon their hearts.

In 1955 Dr. C. Walton Lillehei conceived the novel idea that the defects inside the heart might be corrected if in some way the heart and lungs could be by-passed, so that the heart could actually be opened and repaired under direct vision.

Extracorporeal circulation was developed. This phrase means that the blood is purified and circulated outside of the body. In the normal circulation flow, all impure blood returns to the heart by way of two large veins, the superior and inferior venae cavae, which empty into the right auricle. The blood goes to the right ventricle which pumps it to the lungs. The purified blood returns to the left auricle and goes into the left ventricle which pumps it through the aorta to the entire body.

Extracorporeal circulation is accomplished in this procedure: After the chest has been opened, tubes are placed in the superior and inferior venae cavae. Through these tubes all the impure blood is siphoned off and directed to an oxygenator. The oxygenator is a large glass cylinder in which discs rotate. The lower half of each disc dips into the blood and, as it turns, picks up a film of blood over which a constant stream of oxygen is directed. By the time the blood has passed by about seventy-five discs it has been purified. The purified blood is then returned to the body by an electrical pump which forces the blood through a tube placed in one of the large branches of the aorta. This is a remarkable process. The heart and lungs are by-passed and are free of blood so that it is possible to open the heart and under direct vision, looking right at it, repair the defects. Be not deceived, use of the heart-lung oxygenator or extracorporeal circulation is not as simple as it sounds. Eight to ten pints of blood must be obtained for each operation to prime the pump and the oxygenator. The blood must be heparinized, or rendered incoagulable, during the operation, and as soon as the operation is finished, coagulability of the blood must, of course, be carefully restored. An infinite number of details require exacting attention.

Today the heart defects commonly referred to as the tetralogy of Fallot are corrected by open heart surgery. Through an incision in the right ventricle the obstruction to the pulmonary blood flow is removed and the hole between the two ventricles is closed with a patch of plastic material, called Ivalon. The operation is not an easy one nor without danger, but it does give the child a good chance to live a normal life. To perfect the technique, which is severely difficult and demanding, a surgical team which contemplates doing open heart surgery on children first performs the operation on dogs innumerable times until every single detail has been mastered. The newer operation is attended with more danger than the shunt operations devised originally, but it does have the advantage of giving the child a better chance for a normal life. For this reason parents are usually willing to accept the greater surgical risk.

HOLES IN THE HEART OR SEPTAL DEFECTS

The heart is divided into four chambers. The right auricle is separated from the right ventricle by the tricuspid valve; the left auricle is separated from the left ventricle by the bicuspid or mitral valve. Between the auricles and between the ventricles are walls or septa. A hole in the wall between the auricles is called an interauricular septal defect and a hole in the wall between the ventricles is known as an interventricular septal defect.

A septal defect, unless very tiny, is particularly serious because the left side of the heart is stronger than the right. Consequently with each heartbeat some blood is pumped through the defect into the right auricle or ventricle. To pump this "escaped" blood to the lungs, plus the blood returning from the body, obviously puts an extra strain on the right side of the heart. Furthermore, the increased amount of blood returning from the lungs puts a strain on the left side of the heart. Obviously, therefore, over a period of years the heart slowly wears out because of excessive work.

Symptoms depend entirely upon the size of the defect. The average child with an opening the size of a nickel in the auricular wall or the size of a dime in the ventricular wall is apt to develop symptoms between the ages of two to five years. A murmur caused by the rush of blood through the abnormal openings will be heard just to the left of the breast bone. The child will tire more readily than normal and an X-ray picture of the chest will show that the heart is somewhat enlarged.

During recent years surgeons have devised all sorts of operations for the blind closure of such defects. By blind closure is meant sewing up the hole while the heart is beating. The surgeon introduced a finger into the chamber, identified the hole, and then tried to close it with blindly placed stitches. The results of these operations were poor. Only if the defect were in a select spot would it be possible to effect a satisfactory closure. Attempts to close defects between the ventricles were almost universally unsuccessful.

More recently auricular septal defects have been and still are being closed under direct vision with the aid of hypothermia, that is, reduction of the patient's temperature to well below normal. The lower a person's temperature is, the lower is his metabolism, and therefore less oxygen is consumed. In fact, with each degree centigrade of reduction in temperature, the oxygen requirements fall seven per cent. The lower the temperature, the lower is the metabolism of such important organs as the heart and the brain. It has been found, however, that a person's temperature may not safely be reduced below approximately 82 to 85 degrees Fahrenheit. At normal temperature blood circulation may safely be interrupted approximately four minutes without damage to important tissues. Under hypothermia the circulation may safely be stopped for seven minutes. Although the process of reducing a child's temperature sounds frightening, it is safe so long as the temperature is not lowered beyond 82 degrees Fahrenheit.

The child is first anesthetized, then placed in slush ice water. One electrical thermometer on a wire is introduced through the mouth into the esophagus, and another is inserted into the rectum. As soon as the temperature has dropped to about 90 degrees Fahrenheit, the operation is begun. The temperature will continue to drift downward another five to seven degrees.

The circulation is stopped and the auricle is opened. The surgeon now has a maximum of seven minutes to close the defect in the auricle. If all goes well the time is adequate. However, if unexpected difficulties arise or unanticipated findings are encountered, there is trouble and lots of it. Therefore, most cardiac surgeons have now discontinued hypothermia as an adjunct for closure of auricular septal defects and they employ extracorporeal circulation which allows leisurely and accurate correction of the defect and of other unsuspected abnormalities.

Interventricular septal defects are universally closed under direct vision with the help of extracorporeal circulation.

ISOLATED PULMONARY VALVULAR STENOSIS

As the term isolated pulmonary valvular stenosis suggests, this congenital deformity is limited to the pulmonary valve. Normally the pulmonary valve is made of three paper-thin, beautifully constructed cusps, which lie adjacent to each other in the pulmonary artery at the point where it emerges from the heart. When the heart beats, the filmy valve collapses and permits blood to flow unimpeded through the pulmonary artery. Immediately after the beat, while the heart is momentarily at rest, the valve cusps instantly fill out and prevent blood from flowing back or regurgitating into the relaxed ventricle. A heart valve is really not too different from any type of commercial valve, and its action is exactly the same. The only difference between the live valve and a hardware-store valve is that the live valve, if free from congenital deformity and from later disease, will function without repair for a hundred years.

Why a specific structure, such as a valve, should be deformed—and often it is the only deformity the child has—remains a puzzling mystery. In isolated pulmonary valvular stenosis or narrowing, the edges of the three cusps are so fused together at their bases that only a tiny hole a few millimeters in diameter remains in the center of the vessel. Obviously, if the cusps are completely fused together, the baby dies at birth. However, if the fusion is minimal, the patient may go through life without any handicap other than a slight harmless murmur. In the majority of cases the diameter of the opening through the stenotic valve is about one-fourth the diameter of the pulmonary artery. As a result of this obstruction the right ventricle is called upon to do the extra work of forcing blood through a small aperture.

Children born with this deformity often have very few symptoms.

A loud murmur, produced by blood being squirted through a small opening, is heard by the physician during a routine physical examination. The murmur, plus enlargement of the heart demonstrated by X-ray pictures, suggests the diagnosis, but catheterization of the heart is indicated and necessary for confirmation and determination of the degree of obstruction.

Catheterization of the heart sounds rather formidable but isn't, and a child old enough to cooperate doesn't even need an anesthetic. A long flexible tube or catheter is inserted into a vein at the elbow and threaded upwards into the heart. When the tube reaches the right ventricle, the ventricular pressure is measured by means of a fine, electronically controlled recording instrument. If pulmonary stenosis exists, pressure in the right ventricle is apt to be high. The catheter is then manipulated until it goes through the narrowed valve into the main pulmonary artery where the pressure is low. The pressure gradient or level between the right ventricle and the pulmonary artery determines the severity of stenosis. Blood pressure of 80 to 100 millimeters of mercury in the right ventricle, and of 10 to 20 millimeters of mercury in the pulmonary artery, indicates a rather severe degree of stenosis, which if not relieved will eventually cause heart failure.

Electrocardiograms, relied upon so extensively in the study of adult heart disease, are equally invaluable in determining a diagnosis of pulmonary stenosis, or narrowing, in a child. The electrocardiogram that shows excessive strain on the right ventricle is another reason for early operation.

Operative correction of this deformity is a satisfactory procedure. There is no set age most suitable for operation because each case is an individual problem. Severe pulmonary stenosis demands immediate operation; the youngest child operated upon for this condition at our hospital was only twenty-three days old, and she survived. Some children because of minimal symptoms are not referred to a heart center for examination before they are ten or twelve years old.

For the operation the child is anesthetized and the temperature reduced to about 85 degrees Fahrenheit. The chest is opened, and the superior and inferior venae cavae are isolated and surrounded with loose tapes. Then the aorta and the right and left pulmonary arteries are similarly isolated. When all is in readiness and everyone at the operating table knows exactly what to do, the tapes on all the isolated large vessels are tightened to stop completely the flow of blood through the heart. The surgeon then has five minutes to open the valve under direct vision.

Through a longitudinal incision in the base of the main pulmonary artery, the valve is exposed and with a scissors the fused valve cusps are separated from each other. The slit in the pulmonary artery is closed, all the tapes are released, and normal circulation is restored. The actual procedure of opening the valve usually takes about two minutes. The only reason for hypothermia, or reducing the patient's temperature, is to allow for longer safe interruption of the circulation, in case more time should be needed for the operation or if some other minor deformity requires correction.

After operation—truly, a rather safe procedure—the heart returns to normal size when restrictions on activity are removed. About six weeks following a successful operation, the youngster shouts and dashes off to play and the parents heave a sigh of great relief.

[The operation sounds simple. It is, but it is the result of years of study, of research, of work with dogs, and finally of precision, teamwork, and ability.—Editor's note.]

TRANSPOSITION OF THE GREAT VESSELS

Two large blood vessels arise from the base of the heart. The pulmonary artery, stemming from the right ventricle, carries unoxygenated blood to the lungs, and the aorta, stemming from the left ventricle, carries oxygenated blood to the entire body.

A few children are born with transposition of these two vessels—the aorta arises from the right ventricle and the pulmonary artery from the left ventricle. Under such circumstances impure blood, returned from the body to the right ventricle, is pumped through the misplaced aorta throughout the body without being oxygenated.

How can a child survive if all the blood by-passes the lungs? This is a reasonable question. Unless the defects or openings are in the walls between the auricles and/or ventricles, the baby dies shortly after birth. A fair amount of blood flows to and fro through these defects and allows for some oxygenation. If the defects are small, the baby may live a few weeks; but if the defects are large, the child may get along fairly well for a number of years.

Obviously these children are very blue. It is amazing how little oxygen a baby requires just to maintain life. A normal person who has always had a full supply of oxygen could not tolerate the reduced amount of oxygen upon which a child with transposition of the great vessels has to live. For normal growth and development, a full quota of oxygen is constantly necessary. The baby, severely blue because of transposition of the great vessels, often remains at birth-weight for months. The only hope for salvage of these children is surgical correction of the misplaced vessels.

It seems quite logical to suggest that all that a surgeon needs to do to correct transposed vessels is to cut them just beyond their origin from the heart, reverse them to their proper position, and sew the ends together. Furthermore, such an operation would seem easy with the aid of the artificial heart-lung machine. The only trouble is that the operation will not work and for this reason: The coronary arteries which nourish the heart muscle normally arise from the aorta just before it emerges from the left ventricle. Unhappily, in case of transposition of the great vessels, the coronary arteries still arise from the aorta although it is attached to the right ventricle. If the surgeon shifted and sewed the vessels into their proper position, the coronary arteries would receive only unoxygenated blood and the oxygen-starved heart muscle would cease to function.

In 1956 Dr. Thomas Baffes had a brilliant idea. Since it is impossible to reverse the position of the great vessels, why not shift the course of the blood returning to the heart? Such an operation was fortunately perfected on dogs. The technique of the operation is sometimes difficult for doctors to understand, and it is less easy to explain to nonprofessional readers. Here, however, are the essentials of the procedure, presented with the hope that they are understandable.

Normally, the superior and inferior venae cavae, the huge veins in the chest, collect all the venous blood returning from the body and empty it into the right auricle. The blood then flows to the right ventricle and is pumped to the lungs. In case of transposition of the great vessels, the impure blood takes the same course to the right ventricle but is pumped to the body through the misplaced aorta. The inferior vena cava carries 60 per cent of the venous blood, the blood in the veins.

Herewith is the principle of the Baffes operation: The course of the venous blood from the inferior vena cava (60 per cent) is shifted to the *left* side of the heart, which in case of transposition of the great vessels pumps blood to the lungs, and the oxygenated blood is shifted from the *right* lung, which carries 60 per cent of the oxygenated blood, to the right side of the heart for distribution throughout the body.

These are the technical steps of the rather difficult and formidable operation by which the objective of changing the course of the circulation is accomplished. One end of a two-inch-long, preserved blood vessel graft is sewed to the inferior vena cava. The pulmonary vein carrying oxygenated blood from the right lung to the left auricle is cut, and to the stump of this vessel on the left auricle, the other end of the graft previously attached to the inferior vena cava is sewn. The long end of the right pulmonary vein carrying oxygenated blood is implanted into the right auricle. By these maneuvers, 60 per cent of the impure blood is shifted to the left side of the heart and pumped to the lungs, and a similar amount of pure blood is shifted to the right side of the heart and pumped throughout the body. It is somewhat difficult to keep all the lefts and rights straight.

The operation is actually a makeshift procedure in that it does not correct malposition of the great vessels nor deformities inside the heart, but it does provide sufficient improvement in oxygenation to permit a fairly happy though restricted life. Life expectancy, obviously, is far from normal.

A three-year-old girl, the second patient operated upon by this procedure at the Children's Memorial Hospital in Chicago, was flown in from Alaska during the summer of 1956. She weighed only twenty-three pounds, was blue as grapejuice, and completely helpless. She survived the operation. The following Christmas her parents sent us a picture showing their daughter pulling a sled through the snow. She now attends public school. This is one story of more than a hundred children who have survived this operation at our hospital.

Numerous attempts to correct completely transposition of the great vessels have been made but to date have failed. Until a better curative operation is devised, we shall have to utilize less than perfect procedures to make life tolerable for those children unfortunately born with transposition of the great vessels.

IN CONCLUSION

The story of surgery for congenital heart disease is a happy and exciting one, written during the past twenty years, but not yet finished. Refinements in diagnosis and technique of surgery constantly demand that each chapter be rewritten at least once a year. Some of the chapters in this story are sad, because so far some congenital defects of the heart cannot be corrected. One of the most distressing tasks that confronts a cardiac surgeon is telling a parent that nothing can be done for his child. Learning that their child has a congenital heart defect, parents will travel long distances to heart centers, and with shining hope in their eyes anticipate that some magic operation will be performed so that their child will be normal. It is a terrible shock to them to find out that some defects cannot be corrected.

Only a few of the common heart defects with which children are born have been reviewed. Actually, at present there are seventeen different and specific congenital heart defects that can be cured or improved by operation. All this progress has been made in twenty years.

So long as we do not know why children are born with deformed hearts and so long, therefore, as we are unable to avoid the misfortunes, surgeons will continue to correct the defects as best they can, while earnestly and untiringly seeking new operations and greater improvements of those already in use.

CHAPTER XVI

The Diet and Heart Disease

ANCEL KEYS, Ph.D.

THE DIET for heart patients, as well as everyone else, should provide good general nutrition, including adequate amounts of proteins, minerals, and vitamins. This is easily achieved by using a wide variety of natural foodstuffs with a minimum of highly processed foods that may contain calories but little else. Sugars and fats have their place in the diet but they are so heavy in calories and low in other nutrients that they are often referred to as "empty calories." Preference should be given to fruits, vegetables, lean meats, sea food, and low-fat milk products such as skim milk and cottage cheese.

Besides these general rules dictated by ordinary nutritional considerations, special dietary considerations apply in heart disease, both for heart patients and for those who hope to avoid heart disease. There is no evidence that heart disease is caused by dietary deficiency except in beriberi heart disease, which is caused by severe and prolonged shortage of thiamine (vitamin B_1). Beriberi in the United States is occasionally seen in chronic alcoholics whose diets are extremely abnormal, but otherwise the condition is rare indeed.

Heart diseases are of many kinds and they have various causes but they all share the common characteristic of an actual or impending reduction in the capacity of the heart to work as a powerful and efficient blood pump. The heart patient, then, should not overstrain his limited capacity and, if possible, should reduce the load of work the heart has to do. The diet is important in this respect as a part of management. A proper diet for the cardiac patient may decrease the load on the heart by reducing the body weight or by aiding in the control of fluid in the body or both.

Heart patients frequently suffer from edema or "dropsy" in which fluid accumulates in the body. The ankles swell, the face may become puffy, and examination may reveal fluid in the abdomen and even in the chest. The patient is in heart failure and the fluid accumulation is both dangerous and uncomfortable. Restricting drinking water is useless as well as being most unpleasant. But restriction of salt in the diet helps because edema fluid is a salt solution and without salt the kidneys excrete the excess water.

The body weight is important because the lower it is, the less effort, and correspondingly less blood circulation, is required to move it around. Many heart patients find that after losing some weight they have far less breathlessness, palpitation, and angina pectoris (chest pain) than before, simply because less effort is required to move a lighter body. Even in rest the circulatory demand of a thin body is less than that of a fat body. Reduction of body fat, too, means less fat in the abdomen and around the heart so the lungs can work better. The fatter the patient, the more possibility there is to improve his status by a reducing diet, but even the patient who is not grossly fat often benefits by reducing to the point of being somewhat underweight.

All such questions of dietary management of the heart patient are the responsibility of the attending physician who should decide whether and how much the dietary calories or salt or both should be reduced. Extreme restriction, starvation, or "salt-free" diets may be dangerous and should not be undertaken except under medical control, especially if anorexigenic, or appetite-killing, drugs or so-called salt substitutes are involved.

The heart patient himself should realize that moderation is the golden rule in the diet and will avoid peculiar diets and excesses of all kinds, including alternating between feast and famine. A large, heavy meal imposes a sudden load on the heart, which must pump extra blood to take care of the digestion. Generally, frequent small meals of a variety of foods is better than overeating at any one meal. Rich foods of high caloric density should give way to foods that contain fewer calories per bite so eating satisfaction can be had even on a reducing diet. This means, again, less sugar and fat, including fatty meats and gravies, and more soups, salads, fruits, and vegetables.

The main concern of this chapter is with the new hopes for the diet as an aid to the prevention of heart disease. From life insurance studies we know that overweight people are unduly prone to develop heart disease as well as to die prematurely from many other ills. The most recent study, a large cooperative effort by the Society of Actuaries published late in 1959, confirms all the previous evidence and shows that persons below the average weight of Americans of the same height and age have better than the average life expectation and that the risk of dying is progressively greater with every increase in relative body weight. Heart disease is a major contributor to these differences in mortality.

A second and newer aspect of the diet in regard to the possible prevention of heart disease is indicated in the recent vast mass of evidence about dietary factors promoting coronary heart disease. This kind of heart disease is the major threat to adult Americans today. Though the clinical condition often appears suddenly, coronary heart disease is generally the result of slowly progressive changes in the arteries involving deposits of cholesterol and other fatty materials derived from the blood. The hope for prevention, or at least delay, of this unhappy development in the arteries resides in two facts. The tendency to form these arterial deposits appears to be related to the concentration of these fatty materials, especially cholesterol, in the blood. This relationship can be shown in animal experiments and there is much evidence that it holds in man as well. The second, and most hopeful, fact is that it is now clear that the character of the diet has a powerful influence on the concentration of these substances in the blood.

PERSPECTIVE IN THE ROLE OF THE DIET

About three-fourths of all heart disease deaths in the United States are now attributed to coronary heart disease and another 15 per cent are ascribed to high blood pressure or hypertensive heart disease, with or without disorder of the coronaries as an associated cause. This means that barely 10 per cent of our heart deaths are caused by all other heart diseases and efforts to control our heart disease problem must give major attention to the coronary and hypertension problems.

Unfortunately, the cause of neither of these conditions is known. Generally agreed is that in most cases we cannot hope to find a single cause and therefore no single item of prevention, including the diet, can be a universal panacea. We must think of a multiplicity of influences rather than one cause that sets in course and promotes the developments that terminate as a coronary occlusion. The same can be said of hypertensive heart disease, the causal influences being different, at least in part, though many patients suffer from both hypertension and coronary heart disease and high blood pressure promotes arterial deposits in animal experiments.

Besides the diet, suspicion is directed towards physical activity (or its lack), and emotional stress or tension, and other factors in the mode of life as being contributors to the development of coronary and hypertensive disease. Of course, heredity plays a role. Some families, which happily are uncommon, are unduly afflicted. To some extent their plight may be related to an unfortunate mode of life which is merely familial, that is to say they have bad habits as family customs, but unquestionably genetic constitution does play a role, sometimes dominant. Finally, aging itself is a factor. Blood pressure and deposits in the arteries tend to increase with age, but we may take hope in the fact that this age trend by no means proceeds at the same pace in all persons and may, we trust, be slowed by suitable alterations in the mode of life.

All this means that the diet as a possible factor in the prevention of heart disease must be viewed in perspective as only one influence, albeit perhaps a major one. We may hope that the application of what is already known about the diet, and the knowledge that is rapidly accumulating from research, will be of real value in prevention in that it should reduce the chance of developing heart disease. But it would be wrong to expect that the diet can ever confer absolute protection such as we have from smallpox by vaccination. Moreover, coronary heart disease is usually the end result of silently progressive alterations in the arteries, changes that began years or decades before the clinical disorder is recognizable. Even though the diet may be able to slow or stop further deposits in the arteries, it may be unable to reverse damage already done, damage which may be enough to afford a basis for the clinical disease when other precipitating factors are added.

DRUGS VERSUS THE DIET

In these days of spectacular developments of new drugs both physicians and the general public are apt to seek miracles, or at least to ask in drugs an easy way to avoid the thought and effort required for dietary adjustment. Diets are proposed for the correction of obesity and for the control of cholesterol in the blood. Why not use drugs for these purposes? There are drugs that depress the appetite and lately many preparations are offered in the hope they may help reduce the blood cholesterol.

The fact is that both obesity and cholesterol control, to be effective, must be maintained as lifelong measures; we are not concerned here with merely reducing weight and cholesterol for a few weeks or months. If drugs are to be relied on for these purposes, the user must be prepared to keep on using them indefinitely. None of these drugs can be guaranteed to be free of undesirable side effects, especially with long-continued dosage. Certainly the appetite depressants, including the amphetamines, cannot be recommended in the long run, though in some cases the physician may turn to them as a temporary aid in establishing a new dietary pattern for his patient. Drugs that may interfere with cholesterol in the body are too new to evaluate either their safety or their efficacy, but if they do have an effect on the blood cholesterol level it is probable that they seriously derange other and necessary chemical processes in the body.

In a different class are preparations that are not really drugs but are really special dietary items sold in drug stores. Indigestible "bulk formers" are sold to give a sense of fullness in eating; much the same effect can be had at far less cost from foods of low caloric density with high fiber or cellulose content which also have some nutrient value in the vitamins and minerals they contain. Fancy preparations of unsaturated fats to be taken as "medicine" to control cholesterol are, in fact, extremely expensive competitors of the simple cooking and salad oils available at every grocer's shop. Often they contain other ingredients added to the basic simple vegetable-seed oil, but these—pyridoxine, lecithin, alpha tocopherol, and so on—have not been shown to have any useful effect.

Finally, special margarines to replace butter or ordinary margarine for the control of blood cholesterol may be found in drug stores. Some of these are, in fact, a step in the right direction because they contain less saturated fat, and when used to replace butter they do tend to lower the blood cholesterol to a limited extent. The only objection to them is the exorbitant price asked. It is expected, however, that these margarines will soon be marketed in food shops at a more reasonable price. Their cost of production should be little different from that of conventional margarines and they are at least as safe.

LIMITATIONS OF KNOWLEDGE—WHAT DO WE DO NOW?

Throughout this chapter we must emphasize the present limitations of knowledge. We know that overweight is associated with an increased risk of heart disease. It is possible, however, that some of this bad prognosis is not due simply to being overweight from overeating. People who tend to be overweight may also be prone to heart disease just because that is the way they are constituted. Or it may be that some overweight people are inclined to eat a bad diet in other respects besides simply eating too much. These and other considerations preclude a final conclusion that, in general, overweight causes heart disease which may be prevented merely by reducing the diet and the body weight. But the evidence is strong enough to make a good argument for practical action, particularly when we often see a fall in blood pressure in the reduced person, and when we also know that the overweight heart patient is benefited by reduction.

Much the same holds for control of the cholesterol level in the blood. We know that persons with high blood cholesterol levels are unduly prone to develop coronary heart disease, we know that the cholesterol level can be reduced by dietary means, and we know that the diet can raise the blood cholesterol and produce arterial damage in experimental animals. There is no final proof that changing the diet in adult men so as to lower the blood cholesterol will actually provide a significant measure of protection. Again, we must admit limitations to ultimate knowledge. But the argument is strong and no risk is involved in making the practical decision to use modern dietary knowledge to control the blood cholesterol.

OVERWEIGHT AND OBESITY

Obesity means fatness and the common understanding is that an obese person is overly fat. It is possible to judge roughly whether you are fat, and if so to what extent, merely by visual inspection aided by pinching up skinfolds here and there on the body. What you feel in a skinfold is primarily the thickness of the fat under the skin and it should be noted that about half the total fat of the body is in this subcutaneous layer. This fat under the skin can be measured by special methods but in general the attempt is made to judge fatness indirectly from the body weight.

Table 1 lists the average body weights of Americans of different ages and heights as found many years ago in life insurance examinations. A more elaborate form of this table is still commonly used to judge overweight; if you are twenty pounds over the tabular value, you are said to be overweight by twenty pounds and the inference is that your body contains that much more fat than the average. Actually, this is a highly questionable guide in all but gross departures from the average weight. You may be overweight because of large muscular development, from having a large and heavy bony skeleton, from being full of excess fluid (edema), or any combination of these with or without excess body fat.

The life insurance companies have recognized the limitation of their tables of average weights in regard to application to persons who have different body builds. Revised tables have been suggested in which persons of "heavy" or "large frame" are allowed to be about 8 per cent heavier than those of "medium frame," while persons of "small frame" size have to be proportionately lighter to correspond with the average figures listed in Table 1. But these tables with allowances for frame size have no basis in actual measurements and there is no agreed system for judging frame size.

TABLE 1

Average Body Weight, in Pounds

(nude or in minimal underclothing, according to height and age in years)

MEN

Age	Height in inches without shoes							
	60	62	64	66	68	70	72	74
20	109	115	122	130	138	146	156	166
25	114	119	127	135	143	151	163	174
30	118	123	130	138	146	156	168	180
35	120	125	132	140	150	160	172	185
40	123	128	135	143	153	164	176	190
45	125	130	137	145	155	166	178	192
50	126	131	138	146	156	167	180	194
55	127	132	139	148	158	168	181	195

WOMEN

Age								
	56	58	60	62	64	66	68	70
20	103	107	111	117	124	132	139	148
25	106	110	114	120	127	135	143	150
30	109	113	117	124	130	138	146	153
35	112	116	120	126	134	142	150	156
40	116	120	125	131	138	146	154	160
45	119	123	129	134	142	149	157	164
50	122	126	131	137	144	153	161	169
55	122	126	131	137	145	155	163	170

It will be noted in Table 1 that the average weight at given height increases with age. The Metropolitan Life Insurance Company has decided that there is no good biological excuse for this progressive weight gain long after true body growth has finished. Noting the adverse mortality experience associated with increasing weight, they have proposed that *desirable* weights are simply the averages found for men and women at age twenty-five. In essence, you may use Table 1 as a guide to desirable weight by using only the data for age twenty-five, no matter what your age. It should be noted, of course, that this still does not answer the question as to what kind of tissue makes up your body weight.

Many champion athletes are overweight, according to any of the above systems of tabular weights, but they are decidedly not fat and would be foolish to try to lose weight by going on a diet. On the other hand, many a sedentary businessman or idle housewife is excessively fat in spite of not being overweight because they are deficient in muscle which they have replaced by fat. So read the scales and the tables with understanding, and if your own weight is not grossly out of line with the tables, use other criteria before you decide whether you are fat or thin.

Body weight changes are far more useful than gross body weight. If you have gained a good deal of weight lately, it is a safe bet that you have accumulated fat unless there is reason to suspect that edema is involved, in which case you certainly need personal medical attention. And if you are on a reducing diet, you can watch the scales to know how well you are succeeding. Here again we must mention fluid in the body because this may vary a few pounds from time to time, but it is soon self-correcting. In other words, if you go on a reducing diet and lose ten pounds or nothing in a week, do not be too elated or depressed; variations in body hydration are common right after a major change in the diet but water balance is usually back to normal in ten days or so.

INSURANCE DATA ON OVERWEIGHT

For many years life insurance company studies on the experience with their policy holders have repeatedly shown that overweight, as defined by their tables, is associated with increased risk of death. In general, the total mortality rate is increased by 40 to 50 per cent for persons who are 25 per cent or more overweight, and the insurance experience certainly justifies the practice of charging extra insurance premiums to persons who are greatly overweight. The most recent study, summarized below in Table 2, indicates that mortality advances with every increase in body weight, beginning with persons who are actually underweight according to the old standards.

TABLE 2

Relative Mortality Rates of Life Insurance Policy Holders

Without Known Impairments to Health

(classed according to relative body weight at time of policy issue)

Ages are at time of issue of policy. Mortality rates are for the period 1–19 years after issue of policy. For each sex and age class the mortality rate is expressed as a percentage of the rate for the persons classed as slightly underweight or average weight. Computed from data in *Build and Blood Pressure Study,* Vol. 1, 1959, Society of Actuaries.

RELATIVE BODY WEIGHT	AGES 15–39		AGES 40–69	
Class	Men	Women	Men	Women
Markedly underweight	94	94	96	98
Slightly underweight or average	100	100	100	100
Slightly overweight	119	112	113	122
Moderately overweight	136	122	124	143
Markedly overweight	166	149	145	147

From the discussion on overweight and obesity, above, it is obvious that these data are inadequate to answer the question as to what extent overeating and obesity are responsible for the bad mortality record of overweight persons. The insurance companies have records of a few grossly overweight persons who reduced, and thereby qualified for lower insurance premiums, and these show a more favorable mortality experience than their counterparts who did not reduce their overweight.

The insurance records, useful as they are, must be questioned on the ground not only that they do not directly concern obesity, but also that they have no information about the body weight after the insurance policy has been issued. Clinical studies, however, including comparisons of coronary patients with healthy people and follow-up studies after the clinical appearance of coronary heart disease, give some support to the insurance company conclusions.

Some, but not all, clinical studies find that coronary patients are relatively heavier than the healthy population while other investigators find a somewhat elevated frequency of obesity, judged from simple inspection, in their patients. All sources, however, agree that coronary heart disease often occurs in persons who are not obese or who are actually thin. Simply being thin, then, is small guarantee of safety from the disease.

Curiously, two major researches agree that when coronary heart disease develops, the patients who are fat have a better prognosis than those who are thin. Their mortality is less in the critical first month after an occlusion and the five-year and ten-year survival rates are also better. Perhaps this is because the fat patient has more possibility of improving his status by dieting than the thin patient; he has more fat to lose, more load he can take from his damaged heart.

CORRECTION OF OBESITY

There are plenty of good books on reducing, and this is not the place to go into practical details. Basically, all obesity is the result of eating more food than needed to balance the energy expenditure of the body. The imbalance may be the result of grossly excessive eating or underexpenditure of energy, or both; correction must reverse the picture.

We all know about fat people who claim to eat very little and who blame their shape on a "super-efficient digestion" or state that "everything I eat turns to fat." There is no such thing as a "super-efficient digestion"; all normal people digest and utilize around 95 per cent of the food value eaten. But it is true that many obese people do not eat a great deal. In these cases investigation shows that lack of physical activity is the major factor. Fat people are usually physically indolent, partly because that is their disposition, partly because being fat discourages exercise.

The ideal reducing program attacks the problem from both sides—less food and more exercise, preferably so adjusted that weight is lost at a steady but moderate rate, ten pounds a month or less. Crash reducing diets are ill-advised, as are diets made up of only a few food items. The successful reducer is the person who learns a new way of living—eating and exercise—while reducing and can therefore continue in this reformed manner indefinitely. In any case, it is important to have medical advice before going on any reducing program aimed at losing more than a few pounds.

Psychological factors are involved in most cases of gross obesity. This does not necessarily mean any serious emotional problem. People often overeat from boredom and in a subconscious substitution of eating pleasure for other satisfactions. Some men overeat to express appreciation of their wives' efforts in the kitchen. Some women overeat for the same reason—having prepared a good meal they feel they ought to compliment their own cooking—or they set an example to encourage their children to "clean the plate." Much overeating is an automatic result of the fact that entertaining and being entertained too often centers on eating because people cannot think of other things to do.

Many people overeat because it often relieves tensions and promotes sleep. It is difficult to concentrate on your worries while eating a good meal, and a full stomach has a tranquilizing and soporific effect. Some overeating is promoted by the subconscious mental association between eating and health. We all know that sick people often cannot eat, and we often use the expression, "You are not eating. Don't you feel well?" Years of childhood conditioning frequently have their effect on the attitude toward eating later in life. Hidden in memory is the echo of the admonition, "Eat up. You want to be strong, don't you? You don't want to be sick, do you? Eat up!"

The first step toward successful reducing is a clear realization as to why you want to reduce, coupled with a firm resolution to go through what may be an ordeal at times. The question should be asked, why and how did you get so fat? If you were not always fat, you must have changed your manner of life, diet or exercise, or both, so as to put you in your present state. Did you begin to eat different foods, have more frequent snacks, take larger portions? Did you slacken off on exercise, give up sports, take to using the car when you might readily have walked?

Your problem is to reverse the process that made you fat, and a real change in your mode of life will be involved. Successful reducing is not simply a question of eating a special diet for a few weeks or months. You want to lose your excess fat and not regain it, so when you start on your program you should be prepared to give up some of your former habits forever. You must be psychologically ready for successful reducing, so think it through before you get involved in a half-hearted attempt which may do your self-esteem and will power real harm if you fail.

STAYING SLIM

Staying slim is often more difficult than simple reducing. If you have been fat and have reduced, constant vigilance is needed to adhere firmly to your new mode of life, to prevent slipping back into your old ways. Here the bathroom scales, together with a faithful record of your weight every week, are invaluable. Variations of up to three or four pounds may be neglected but five pounds or more, especially if this gain holds or increases for two successive weeks, means the necessity for diet and exercise adjustment.

Most people who become seriously obese show the tendency at an early age and often have a lifelong problem to reduce and stay reduced. The person who, at the age of thirty, say, is still relatively slim, finds it much easier to stay that way or, if he does get fat, to reduce permanently.

As people proceed through life beyond the twenties, they find it increasingly easier to avoid real exercise, and higher incomes tempt one to have more and especially richer food. It is not a bad idea to say to oneself that getting fat and soft is to grow older and then to resolve not to grow older. Here again the bathroom scales and a record is a constant reminder. Do not allow yourself to get fat; but if you are fat, resolve to correct this so as to look better, feel better, and live longer.

THE CORONARY PROBLEM

Coronary heart disease is sometimes called arteriosclerotic heart disease because the primary disorder is in the arteries. The heart muscle depends for its nourishment and "breathes" through the coronary arteries that form a crown around the heart before they plunge down into the heart muscle to bring fresh blood to every cell. Any interference with this blood supply is dangerous and can be quickly fatal. Such interference can be produced by a form of arteriosclerosis called atherosclerosis in which there are deposits of cholesterol and associated cellular changes in the wall of the artery and by blood clots, or coronary thrombosis, which block the blood passage. These clots or thrombi generally form only in an artery damaged with arteriosclerosis.

The facts leading to the belief that a large measure of prevention of coronary heart disease can be achieved by dietary regulation may be summarized as follows:

1) The frequency of coronary heart disease varies greatly between populations that eat different amounts and kinds of fats. Coronary heart disease is a minor problem among populations whose diets contain relatively little of the common meat and dairy fats that bulk so large in the current American diet. Such populations are not all in "underdeveloped" countries and they may have good health in other respects, too.

2) These differences between populations are not dependent on climate or race. There is a great difference in the frequency of the disease between rich and poor Italians in Naples and Neopolitans living in Boston, between rich and poor Spaniards in Madrid, between economic classes of people in Guatemala. Japanese in Southern California are like other Californians in the frequency of the disease but are more often affected than their semi-Americanized relatives in Hawaii who, in turn, have far more coronary heart disease than men in Japan.

3) These differences between populations are not explained by personal habits such as the habitual use of tobacco or alcohol. Many of the populations who suffer relatively little coronary heart disease contain plenty of men who are heavy smokers or drinkers or both. If tobacco or alcohol have any effect, this does not seem to be primary.

4) Coronary heart disease is much more common in populations in whom the average blood contains large amounts of cholesterol than among those whose blood cholesterol levels are relatively low.

Investigations embracing more than a score of populations around the world suggest that the frequency of early, severe coronary disease in a population is closely proportional to the average serum cholesterol concentration in the population.

5) Follow-up studies in the United States clearly show that men with high concentrations of cholesterol in the blood are much more prone to develop coronary heart disease in the next few years and, in fact, the risk of coronary heart disease is directly related to the blood cholesterol level.

6) The serum cholesterol level in man rapidly responds to changes in dietary fat, falling when meat and dairy fats are reduced, rising when they are replaced in the diet, even when calories, proteins, and vitamins are kept constant. Some vegetable oils have no such effect and may even reduce the serum cholesterol.

7) Animals fed diets that raise the cholesterol level in the blood serum develop disease in the coronary arteries, and the extent of the disease tends to parallel the serum cholesterol level. Return to a more favorable diet restores the cholesterol level to normal and the artery disease tends to regress.

8) Populations whose diets are changed in regard to fat content have been reported subsequently to show important differences in the frequency of coronary heart disease. Examples are European countries during and after World War II, immigrants into Israel, Japanese moving from Japan to Hawaii to California. No exceptions have been reported.

All of this does not deny influences other than the diet, but it is clear that the cholesterol level in the blood is important and that this level is sensitive to the diet, particularly the fats in the diet.

CHOLESTEROL AND OTHER LIPIDS IN THE BLOOD

Cholesterol is a waxy material, soluble in ether or gasoline like the true fats and other lipids. It is not poisonous, but it is so stable that once it is deposited in the walls of the arteries it tends to stay there. It creates a mechanical problem by its mere presence and stimulates the adjacent cells of the artery wall to build up a kind of scar tissue which, in turn, creates further difficulties, encroaching on the space for the blood to flow and forming irregularities in the diameter of the lumen of the artery.

Cholesterol is carried in the blood, which is a watery medium, yet it is not soluble in water. Actually, there is little if any plain cholesterol in the blood; it is combined with proteins and fats in so-called giant molecules, the lipoproteins, which are water-soluble. And this also explains how water-insoluble fats can be carried in solution in the blood. The significant point is that cholesterol is an essential part of the lipoproteins—it is needed to form the combination that puts fats into a water-soluble form. Cholesterol, therefore, is not an abnormal or useless substance in the blood but plays a necessary role in making it possible to transport and use fats in the body.

The whole story of what happens to fats from the time they are eaten until they are burned in the body to provide useful energy is complicated and many details are still unknown, but the main features show how cholesterol fits into the picture. First, after we eat fats they are absorbed into the blood, causing the plasma, the liquid part of the blood, to turn cloudy or, if there is much fat, opaque and creamy. The plasma at this stage is an emulsion like milk, with countless tiny droplets of fat suspended in it. The fat cannot be used by the cells of the body in this form, and anyway there is a temporary surplus of fuel after a meal. But after a few hours the plasma becomes clear again, not because the fat has been burned up but because the liver has been busy.

Much fat can be stored as such in the liver, and this is what happens, temporarily, to a good deal of the fat we absorb. This gets the fat out of the way but it does not solve the problem of utilizing it, of providing the fat as a steady supply of fuel to the tissues all over the body. One answer would be to put fat back into the blood but in solution, not in suspension. And so lipoproteins are formed and released into the blood. The net effect is an increase in the amount of cholesterol in the blood. If there is any shortage of cholesterol, the liver promptly makes as much as needed, and some of the fat, after being broken down part way, can be used for this synthesis of cholesterol. As for the protein needed to make the lipoproteins, this is normally at hand.

Lipoproteins are useful in transporting fat in the body but they also create a new problem. The fats in the lipoproteins are valuable fuels, but when they are burned the protein and cholesterol in these lipoprotein molecules remain. The proteins present no problem; they can replace the proteins lost from the cells by "wear and tear," they are readily burned as fuel, and, in any case, they are water-soluble and hence not liable to pile up as deposits. But the cholesterol cannot be so burned and it is a water-insoluble remnant, useless or worse. It is not surprising, then, that some of the cholesterol tends to be deposited in the tissues it finds itself in, particularly in the intima of the arteries.

The liver, which so obligingly makes cholesterol to match the amount of fat to be converted into lipoproteins, also is efficient in disposing of excess cholesterol by excreting it in the bile both as cholesterol and in the slightly altered form of the bile salts. Aside from the occasional danger of forming gallstones (cholesterol is a major constituent of gallstones), this is a satisfactory means of disposal, but the cholesterol must be in the liver to be handled in this way; cholesterol elsewhere in the body has to be brought back to the liver and this is not easy because, again, of the problem of water insolubility.

Of course the cholesterol concentration in the blood, even its average over the years, is not the sole factor in the production of atherosclerosis. Local abnormalities in the structure of the arterial wall or in the way in which the arteries branch may favor the formation of atherosclerosis even if the concentration of cholesterol in the blood is not very high. Such abnormalities may be inherited or may be produced, by causes unknown, during early development. If they are present, they increase the danger associated with any given level of cholesterol in the blood. Then, too, a severe degree of atherosclerosis, with much cholesterol deposited in the artery wall, does not always produce coronary heart disease, while on the other hand a single spot in a strategic location may be the site of a fatal clot. None of this lessens the importance of atherosclerosis or the cholesterol in the blood that promotes it.

People differ in their serum cholesterol levels even on the same diet. There is a general tendency for the level to rise from youth until the fifties or sixties and then to decline at still older ages. It is interesting that this age trend in the blood has a counterpart in the arteries where the rate of development of atherosclerosis is similarly related to age, rising from early adulthood until late middle age with not much new atherosclerosis developing thereafter. This suggests that as we get older, dietary control becomes increasingly important, at least until the years of old age.

Besides this general age trend, there is a great deal of variability between individuals of the same age. If you are forty years old and living on an ordinary American diet, the chances are that you have a blood serum cholesterol concentration between 220 and 270 milligrams per 100 cubic centimeters, but you may be in the 300-plus class or, on the other hand, among the fortunate few with an average value less than 200. There is no explanation at present for these differences in most cases. It is known that both diabetes and deficient function of the thyroid gland raise the cholesterol, while excessive activity of the thyroid sometimes produces unusually low levels. But attempts to regulate the cholesterol with thyroid hormone are both unsuccessful and undesirable unless there is real evidence of thyroid disorder.

So the importance of the diet is not the same for everyone. From cholesterol measurements in the blood of thousands of persons all over the world, we know that not many adult Americans have serum cholesterol values as low as the averages in populations who have relatively low susceptibility to coronary heart disease. But some Americans are in this class and we see no reason why these individuals should change their present diet. Your physician can arrange for a blood analysis and advise you. Of course, your serum cholesterol concentration is far from being an infallible indicator of your coronary future. You must not let your life insurance lapse just because your report comes back "cholesterol 180 mg.%." Similarly, the finding of a high value is not necessarily a cause for alarm, although it may properly produce determination to do something about it.

The cholesterol values of individuals vary spontaneously from time to time, even when the diet is constant. It has been suggested that emotional strain may have something to do with these variations, but in any case it must be realized that a single blood cholesterol measurement does not necessarily give a precise picture of the average habitual level.

Physicians as well as patients and the general public frequently ask what should be considered the "normal" concentration of cholesterol in the blood. It is not enough to decide this on the basis of a series of measurements on persons who are, at the time, clinically healthy. Many such persons, in the United States at least, already have severe coronary atherosclerosis which is symptomless and invisible but will sooner or later produce clinical coronary heart disease.

If we judge from follow-up studies of middle-aged men whose blood serum cholesterol was measured while they were clinically healthy, we must conclude that values of over 260 milligrams of cholesterol per 100 milliliters of serum are dangerous and that values less than 220 are associated with a less than average risk of future heart attacks. If we study the cholesterol values in populations that suffer little from coronary heart disease, we conclude that the lower the cholesterol value the better in this respect. And if we study patients who have the disease, we find that relatively few of them have cholesterol values as low as 220. From these considerations, and the data on the cholesterol values in populations at different ages, we can arrive at rough estimates as to *desirable* cholesterol levels. These are summarized in Table 3.

TABLE 3

Suggested Desirable and Undesirable Levels of Total Cholesterol
(in milligrams per 100 ml. of blood as measured by reliable methods)

No distinction is made as to sex, though it appears that high cholesterol levels in women may take longer than in men to do damage to the arteries.

AGE	DESIRABLE	UNDESIRABLE
Under 25 years	Under 190	Over 220
25–40 years	Under 210	Over 240
Over 40 years	Under 220	Over 250

There are arguments as to which method of blood analysis best reveals the threat of future coronary heart disease. We can measure the total fats, the total cholesterol, or the total lipoproteins in the blood; we can estimate the lipoprotein fractions separately or the cholesterol in the separate fractions. Which method is most likely to single out the persons who are in the greatest danger, and, therefore, in most need of such prophylactic and corrective measures as can be applied? This question has produced a vast deal of heated debate, but it now appears that several of these methods differ relatively little in their predictive value. They all have high statistical value in comparing groups of people; no particular measurement, or even all methods put together, is very reliable in predicting the fate of an individual. We are personally inclined to think that the measurement of cholesterol in the beta lipoprotein fraction of the blood serum is a little more informative than the others. But this complicated and expensive procedure is at most only a trifle better than the simple total cholesterol measurement. No other method, including the use of the ultracentrifuge, has been shown to be more reliable than the plain cholesterol measurement in spite of the propaganda from some laboratories which offer commercial analyses and promise a report on the "atherogenic index."

BLOOD CHOLESTEROL AND SOME DIETARY COMPONENTS

Cholesterol itself is contained in all fatty foods of animal origin, especially in egg yolks, but ordinarily the cholesterol we ingest in the diet in this way has little or no effect on the cholesterol concentration in the blood of man. When rabbits or chicks are fed cholesterol, the level rises greatly in the blood but man and many other animals, including dogs and rats, are far more able to handle dietary cholesterol. In other words, you can eat eggs even if you are trying to reduce your blood cholesterol, but it may be wise to keep to a limit of 3 or 4 egg yolks a week (in all forms) because of the fats they contain; egg whites may be eaten in any amount.

Substances chemically related to cholesterol, the plant sterols or phytosterols, are contained in some foods, notably vegetable-seed oils. Large amounts of phytosterols in the diet, 15 grams or more daily, may have some cholesterol-depressing effect in the blood but the amount of these substances in foods are so small that they may be ignored.

Because some populations with a low incidence of coronary heart disease eat little meat, it has been suggested that a high protein diet may promote the disease. More critical study shows there is no real evidence for this idea and that the low-protein diets in question are more remarkable in being low in fats, which would explain the low serum cholesterol values and infrequency of heart attacks observed in those populations. Experimental variations in the protein level of the diet over a range wider than encountered by ordinary Americans have no effect on the serum cholesterol if the diet is otherwise constant. However, the mistake may be made of believing that a high protein diet is only achieved by gorging on meat; such a diet is really a high fat diet. The blood cholesterol level will tend to be high on such a diet not because of the protein but as a result of the fat in the diet.

Vitamins and minerals in the diet are important in many ways, and accordingly many investigations have sought to find effects of these nutrients on the blood cholesterol level. Except in some highly artificial situations with laboratory animals, all of these studies have been negative with one exception. Nicotinic acid, the antipellagra vitamin, lowers the serum cholesterol level when taken in colossal doses, hundreds of times the vitamin requirement. Such dosages have undesirable side effects but they are prescribed by some physicians who believe it so essential to lower the blood cholesterol level that they are willing to use almost any method that is not clearly dangerous. It is not advisable to try this treatment except under the guidance of a physician. In any case dietary nicotinic acid or ordinary supplements bought at the drug store have no effect.

BLOOD CHOLESTEROL AND DIETARY FATS

The main interest in the character of the diet in regard to coronary heart disease is in the fats. Formerly, fats were dismissed as merely sources of calories, but lately they are in the center of nutritional interest. It is now evident that populations subsisting on low-fat diets are singularly protected from the high frequency of coronary heart disease suffered by populations such as that of the United States who get around 40 per cent, or more, of their total calories from fats. In general, it seems that the average serum cholesterol level and the frequency of coronary heart disease in populations are directly related to the fat content of the diets, but there are some complications. In rural Greece and Dalmatia the diet is fairly high in fat, up to 35 per cent of total calories, but coronary heart disease is much less common than in this country or even than in Finland or Britain where fats provide only slightly more than 35 per cent of the calories. But in all of these countries the serum cholesterol values are more or less parallel to the coronary disease frequency.

The explanation requires consideration of the different kinds of fats and their chemical composition. All fats are triglycerides, that is, compounds of three fatty acid molecules with a glycerine molecule, and we now know that the effects of dietary fats on the blood cholesterol level are due to the fatty acids. There are many different kinds of fatty acids but a classification may be made according to their degree of saturation.

In some fatty acids the chain of carbon atoms in the molecule is fully saturated with attached hydrogen atoms, the chain being an uninterrupted sequence of $CH_2CH_2CH_2CH_2$. . . . These are called saturated fatty acids; they are particularly abundant in butter, in milk fat in general, and the fats of ordinary meats. If two hydrogen atoms are missing from this carbon chain, so that we have $CH_2CHCHCH_2$ . . . , there is one point of unsaturation, one double bond, and we have a mono-ene, or singly unsaturated fatty acid. Oleic acid, so-called because it is the main fatty acid in olive oil, is the most common example. If there are two or more such double bonds in the fatty acid, it is called a polyene; it is poly-unsaturated. Linoleic acid, abundant in most vegetable-seed oils, is an important example of a fatty acid with two points of unsaturation or two double bonds. Fish oils contain fatty acids with five or more double bonds.

Hydrogenated fats, such as in margarines and solid vegetable shortenings, are made by treating vegetable oils to force hydrogen atoms into the places of unsaturation in the fatty acids. Most of the linoleic acid is converted into oleic acid in this way and some of the oleic acid, too, picks up a pair of hydrogens of each molecule and becomes stearic acid, a fully saturated fatty acid. As hydrogen is added the fat becomes more solid so it may be used as a spread and the saturated fats are more stable too, which makes them popular with food manufacturers.

All of this is important because these different kinds of fatty acids have different effects on the blood cholesterol and probably on the development of atherosclerosis and eventual coronary heart disease. Saturated fatty acids in the diet of man raise the blood cholesterol level. Poly-unsaturated fatty acids have an opposing but weaker effect; for example, it takes about two ounces of linoleic acid in the diet to counter the action of one ounce of a saturated fatty acid. Oleic acid, a fatty acid with only one point of unsaturation, has no effect on the serum cholesterol of man and may be exchanged in the diet with equal calories of carbohydrate without altering the serum cholesterol level.

This explains the peculiarity of the Greeks, Dalmatians, and some other groups. Almost all of the fat in their diets is olive oil in which oleic acid makes up about 80 per cent of the fatty acid. Their diets are actually very low in saturated fatty acids so their blood cholesterol levels are correspondingly low. The fat in the usual American diet is largely from meats, dairy products, and hydrogenated margarines and shortenings; we get around 16 to 18 per cent of our total calories from saturated fatty acids. On the Island of Crete the total fat intake approaches our own but only around 5 per cent of the calories in the total diet are supplied by saturated fatty acids. It is not surprising, then, that middle-aged men in Crete average less than 200 milligrams of cholesterol per 100 milliliters of serum while their counterparts in the United States average about 240. And we note, also, that coronary heart disease is not common in Crete.

The lesson from these facts is that the most effective single change of the diet to lower the blood cholesterol is to reduce the intake of saturated fats. This means less fat meat, butter, cream, and other fat-rich dairy products. Poultry is both less fat and the fat in it is less saturated than ordinary meats so it is a good substitute. Fish oils are highly unsaturated so fish is recommended, as are other products of the sea. Table 4 lists the composition of some food fats and oils.

Table 4

Average Fatty Acid Composition of Food Fats and Oils

The figures for butter apply to the fat in milk, cream, cheese, etc. Data from Table 13, pp. 324, 325, in *Eat Well and Stay Well*, by Ancel and Margaret Keys, Doubleday & Company, Inc., by permission.

Item	% Saturated	% Mono-ene	% Poly-ene
OILS			
Coconut	92	6	2
Corn	16	27	57
Cottonseed	28	21	51
Olive	12	80	8
Palm (red)	45	45	10
Peanut	18	56	26
Rape seed	6	68	26
Safflower	12	10	78
Sesame	13	45	42
Soybean	14	30	56
Sunflower	10	18	72
SPREADS AND SHORTENINGS			
Butter	58	39	3
Lard	25–35	50–60	10–18
Margarine, typical	50–64	40	10
Shortening, typical	24–26	61–67	9–13
SEED AND GRAIN FATS			
Barley	13	33	54
Oats	10	59	31
Rice	16	46	38
Rye	21	18	61
Wheat	17	20	63
NUT FATS			
Almond	6	77	17
Brazil	20	56	24
Cashew	14	71	15
Filbert	4	82	10

Pecan	5	79	16
Walnut	5	35	60

COMMON ANIMAL FATS

Beef	48	49	3
Beef heart	45	43	12
Beef liver	40	20	40
Chicken	26	50	24
Egg	31	53	16
Fish	25	–	75
Horse	32	46	22
Lamb	40	55	5
Mutton	50	45	5
Pork	40	48	12
Rabbit (domestic)	40	44	16
Rabbit (wild)	30	32	38
Veal	40	57	3
Venison	66	30	40

MISCELLANEOUS FATS

Cocoa and chocolate	60	38	2
Human body fat	41	46	13

Table 4, and the knowledge that oleic acid is neutral while saturated fatty acids raise the cholesterol level and poly-unsaturated fatty acids have the opposite effect but only about half the potency, is enough to devise effective and palatable diets to control the blood cholesterol. In general, the best plan is to restrict saturated fats as far as possible and to use poly-unsaturated fats fairly liberally for salads and all cooking purposes. The cholesterol response to such a diet is usually measurable in a few days and the full effect is attained in three or four weeks. Thereafter, if the diet is maintained, a new low plateau persists indefinitely. The effect varies between individuals but is largest in those persons who have the highest serum cholesterol values before changing the diet.

DIET CARBOHYDRATES AND BLOOD CHOLESTEROL

Dietary experiments indicate that all carbohydrates are not identical in respect to effect on the serum cholesterol level. When the complex carbohydrates of fruits and vegetables (including beans) are substituted for equal calories of sugar in the diet of man, the serum cholesterol level tends to fall. The decline is not large but it is consistent. Special experiments show that the extra fiber or cellulose in the fruits and vegetables are not responsible but pectin from fruits was found to have a cholesterol-lowering action.

These experimental findings are interesting because they seem to explain the fact that cholesterol levels in some populations are somewhat lower than would be expected from consideration of the dietary fats alone. The diets of these populations are high in fresh fruits and leafy vegetables. Here, then, is more reason to favor an abundance of fruits and vegetables in the diet and to exercise moderation with sugars as well as with other refined foodstuffs.

ALCOHOL AS A PART OF THE DIET

Dietary studies usually neglect alcohol intake, though alcohol supplies 7.1 calories per gram, that is, it is intermediate between carbohydrates and fats in this respect, and many Americans receive from 10 to over 20 per cent of their total calories from this source. Neglect of the caloric contribution of alcoholic beverages can easily wreck a reducing plan. Table 5 gives the caloric values of some common measures of alcoholic beverages.

Apart from the caloric value and therefore significance for body weight control, alcoholic beverages are of interest in other ways in connection with heart disease. Some physicians prescribe small or moderate intakes of alcoholic beverages for cardiac patients in an effort to promote relaxation or to counter the emotional depression found in some patients. The value of alcohol for these purposes may be disputed and its use is a matter of clinical judgment and the personal bias of physician and patient.

TABLE 5

Calories in Common Measures of Alcoholic Beverages

Abbreviated and modified from Table 15 in *Eat Well and Stay Well*, by Ancel and Margaret Keys, published by Doubleday & Company, Inc., by permission.

Item	Alcohol Strength	Unit of Volume	Calories
Beer, 3.2	3.2%	12 oz.	130
Beer, "strong"	6.0%	12 oz.	190
Cocktail, "Manhattan"	60 proof	3 oz.	160
Cocktail, "Martini"	65 proof	3 oz.	170
Whisky, gins, etc.	90 proof	2 oz.	150
Whisky, Bonded	100 proof	2 oz.	170
Wine, dry table	13%	4 oz.	110
Wine, sherry, port	20%	4 oz.	130

Alcohol may reduce the tendency to angina of effort, the chest pain brought on by exercise, but this seems to be merely an analgesic effect and does not imply improvement of coronary circulation. Since angina of effort may be a useful warning of dangerous insufficiency of coronary blood flow, suppression of it by raising the pain threshold could be dangerous.

Years ago it was reported that men dying with chronic alcoholism had less than the average amount of atherosclerosis in their arteries. Other studies have failed to confirm this and, in any case, the general state of undernutrition of such alcoholics might be enough to explain a lack of atherosclerosis without involving the idea of any specific protection from alcohol ingestion.

On a constant diet in which alcohol is substituted for simple carbohydrate to an extent representing 20 per cent of the total calories, the serum cholesterol rises markedly in dogs. In man, dietary experiments show a small but rather consistent rise in the serum cholesterol with this level of alcohol intake, which produces real drunkenness.

More moderate daily alcohol usage, corresponding to one or two strong cocktails a day, does not affect the cholesterol level in man.

The net conclusion about alcohol is that in small or moderate amounts there is no reason to believe it has any effect, pro or con, on the development of coronary heart disease. Very large daily use, corresponding to a third of a bottle of whisky daily, is to be avoided for many reasons of health, including the effect on the blood cholesterol.

HYPERTENSION AND THE DIET—OBESITY

Though little can be said definitely about the cause or causes of most cases of hypertension, there is no doubt that it is often associated with obesity and that a reducing diet generally produces a fall in blood pressure. The fat man who finds he has hypertension is more fortunate than the thin man who has the same elevated level of blood pressure; he can lose weight with a good prospect of correcting his blood pressure or at least of bringing it to a more favorable level.

Severe hypertension, of course, can cause heart disease but there is also evidence that even only moderate elevations of blood pressure carry an added risk of future heart disease. The person who has a blood pressure in the "high normal" range, say 140 over 90, and who is also somewhat fat, runs a double risk. Reduction to the level of being definitely thin is the wise course in such cases.

HYPERTENSION AND THE DIET—SALT

When animals are fed an excessively salty diet for a long time, they develop high blood pressure and it is found that the kidneys have been damaged. This is but one of several reasons for suspecting that a high salt level in the diet may promote hypertension. It is reported that, on the average, persons who always salt their food, even before tasting it, have higher blood pressures than those who taste and then salt and the persons who seldom add salt, even after tasting, have still lower blood pressures.

It is interesting that the frequency of hypertension and its complications is very high in Japan, and blood pressures in the general population there average higher than in other populations. Japanese doctors are inclined to blame this on the high salt content of the Japanese diet. Accurate data are lacking but the daily per capita salt intake in Japan seems to be over two-thirds of an ounce or perhaps twice that in the United States. Soy sauce, which is about a 10 per cent salt solution, is a major contributor to the salty Japanese diet.

These and other indications that salt may promote hypertension by no means prove the case but they do point a justified finger of suspicion. We conclude that moderation in the use of salt is wise. It should be noted that ordinary salt is NaC1 and that it is the Na, or sodium, we are concerned about. Sodium glutamate (sold under various trade names, "Accent," "MSG," "Ajinomoto") cannot be freely substituted for ordinary salt if you are on a low-salt diet. Much of the "salt" in soy sauce used in Japanese and Chinese cooking is in the form of sodium glutamate.

Extremely low-salt diets are sometimes used in the treatment of patients with hypertension. These diets are difficult to prepare and are highly unpalatable to most people. They sometimes produce good results but they should not be used except under medical supervision. Note that for this purpose, that is, in the treatment of severe hypertension, a moderate restriction of salt is not effective; the diet must be really very low in salt and it must be continued that way.

EXERCISE

It is unrealistic to discuss the diet without consideration of exercise. The amount of food in general and of fat in particular in the diet you can eat depends, in part, on the habitual level of exercise. The heart patient may have to avoid exercise because even in rest he is near the limit of his capacity. On the other hand, there is much reason to believe that exercise has some preventive or prophylactic effect against the development of coronary heart disease.

Be guided by your physician if you already have heart disease. If you are not so afflicted, it is well to get plenty of regular exercise. Besides such trivial gestures as a few minutes of calisthenics in the morning or a week-end golf game, more vigorous and prolonged exercise is desirable.

STRESS AND EMOTION

This is not the place to discuss the popular notion that most of our problem of heart disease today is the result of the "stress of modern life." It may well be that emotional stress and tension play an important role in producing both coronary and hypertensive heart disease, but there is nothing approaching good evidence that this is the case.

It is not true that either of these diseases are peculiar afflictions of people who carry the greatest burden of responsibility. But there is much evidence that in many societies the most affluent class suffers most—the class that eats most and most richly, and that has the least exercise.

The point to be emphasized here is that it seems to be both unjustified and unwise to accept the theory that the "stress" of a well-paid job and high responsibility in the community is the main factor in producing heart disease. How can you reduce such stress? A common response is to try to "take it easy," which is apt to mean resting (and not exercising) during the day. And, of course, emphasis on the stress theory would mean that there would be little reason to pay attention to the diet.

PRACTICAL CONCLUSIONS FOR TODAY

Many questions remain. It is not known how much protection the diet can provide against heart disease nor what is precisely the best diet for this purpose. It may be decades before the mechanisms whereby the diet exerts its effects are understood.

Nevertheless, it is clear that the threat of heart disease, and particularly of coronary heart disease, is increased by obesity, by elevated blood pressure, and by high blood-cholesterol concentration. For each of these factors the danger seems to increase in parallel with these characteristics and, moreover, the factors are additive. The worse risk is the fat man with high blood pressure who has a high cholesterol value.

We know that the diet affects the blood cholesterol and obesity and may influence the blood pressure and major factors in these influences have been identified. Dietary adjustments with these points in mind are entirely safe and are not difficult nor unpleasant nor expensive.

One school of thought holds that such dietary adjustments—control of calories, restriction in saturated fats, more liberal use of highly unsaturated fats and, perhaps, more care in the use of salt—are advisable for "high-risk" persons but need not yet be advocated for the general population. High-risk persons are defined as those who have one or more of the following characteristics: overweight, high blood cholesterol value, high blood pressure, a bad family history in regard to coronary heart disease. But do not one or more of these characteristics pertain to most middle-aged Americans today?

A SUMMARY OF FOOD CHOICES

Presuming that the decision is to act on the basis of the information given in this chapter, then practical details of the diet must be considered. These are given at length in the book *Eat Well and Stay Well,* referred to previously. Here space allows only the brief summary of some food choices for the control of the blood cholesterol given in Table 6.

TABLE 6

Choice of Foods for the Control of Blood Cholesterol

Note that the total diet should be made up of a variety of foods and should be adjusted in total calories so as to prevent weight gain or to bring about reduction if a reducing diet is required because of obesity.

UNRESTRICTED FOODS

fruits	buttermilk	beans and other legumes
berries	cottage cheese	fish and shell fish
leafy, flower, and stalk	cereals and breads	egg whites
vegetables	potatoes	true nuts
skim milk	root vegetables	

FOODS IN MODERATION

whole milk	peanuts	rabbit
chicken, other poultry	whole eggs	veal

liquid vegetable oils (*not* including palm or coconut oil)

special margarines (with less than 30 per cent saturated fatty acids and over 12 per cent poly-unsaturated fatty acids)

RESTRICTED FOODS

cream	pork	margarine
high-fat (30% or more fat) cheeses	lard	hydrogenated shortenings
beef	butter	gravies with fats
	ice cream	

CHAPTER XVII

Rest and Activity in Patients with Heart Disease

EMMET B. BAY, M.D.

THE MANAGEMENT of the patient's way of life is still the most important part of his care in all forms of heart disease. All patients with heart disease should be encouraged to be as active as their particular situations will permit. Many studies in normal people and those with heart trouble show that the heart is more efficient when it, as well as the body muscles, are toned up by activity.

This discussion of bodily activity in heart disease will include two large categories: 1) acute conditions in which the need for nearly complete rest is still obvious, and 2) chronic states in which some heart damage exists but in which maximal permissible activity is desirable.

In general, any situation in which something is, or may be, changing in the heart or any of its parts requires bed rest until the process is stationary. Such conditions occur in acute rheumatic fever with heart involvement, subacute bacterial endocarditis, and in acute coronary thrombosis. All these tend to leave scars of varying importance in the heart, which may be reduced by proper treatment of the acute episode, including rest in bed. Other conditions affecting the heart are hyper- or hypothyroidism and anemia. These may require rest at the time they are most active, but successful medical management usually leads to a restoration of the heart to normal without restrictions on the demands made upon it by bodily activity.

A patient with a permanently damaged heart from whatever cause may have to limit his mode of life. This can be better understood and can be more intelligently applied if the function of the normal heart is appreciated. Fortunately, the heart, unlike the liver, has only one job to do: to pump blood. At present it is possible to study the heart as an engineer would examine a water pump. Its work can be measured and expressed in the physical terms of the output of fluid (blood) times the pressure: W (work) = Vp (volume times pressure).

When this concept is applied to man, the proof becomes apparent that a certain amount of work has to be done by the heart day and night to supply oxygen, sugar, and other nutriments to the body at rest. More work has to be done by the heart whenever it is called upon to furnish more of these sources of energy for any one or a combination of activities. These include walking, talking, digestion of food, emotional reactions, exposure to cold and wind, and many others. This ability to respond to increased demands is called the cardiac reserve (graph, page 230). In a healthy young person in good physical condition, the heart can do more than twenty times the work per minute for short intervals than is required just to keep him alive. From the engineering point of view, both the years of trouble-free service and the great flexibility of this pump make the heart a truly marvelous creation.

Chronic heart disease can affect this cardiac reserve in one or both of two ways: 1) by increasing the work of the appropriate part of the heart necessary to maintain life in the basal resting state, and 2) by decreasing the extra work the heart can perform to allow for increased demands. The mechanisms by which it does this vary with the type of heart disease and can be analyzed in an oversimplified way, as follows:

a) Congenital heart disease. Persons born with heart trouble may have narrowings of some places in the pathway through the organ, openings producing shunts in the pathways, or other developmental defects. Some of the shunts reduce the oxygen content of the arterial blood including that part of it going to feed the heart muscle itself. In these cases the heart has to do more work because of the useless additional amount of blood pumped through the by-pass. Also, its supply of extra energy to make the work possible is reduced.

b) Rheumatic heart disease. The scars left in some hearts after acute rheumatic fever has subsided more often affect the mitral and aortic valves on the left side. They may be narrowed as in stenosis, or made leaky as in insufficiency, or both. These deformities may be unimportant or can cause a great increase in the work of the heart at bed rest. They also tend to diminish the ability of the appropriate heart chamber to keep up with the need for more output under conditions of stress. The heart muscle may also be permanently weakened by scarring from rheumatic fever.

c) Coronary heart disease. Coronary heart disease is divided for this discussion of mechanical effects into angina pectoris and coronary thrombosis. Angina pectoris, or pain in the chest, results from a narrowing of one or more branches of the coronary arteries, the vessels that supply the heart muscle itself with blood. When a heart with such arteries has added work to do because of physicial activity or excitement, it cannot get sufficient blood for its needs because of the narrowing, and as a result pain in the chest is produced. This usually subsides quickly when the demand for extra work is eliminated. Coronary thrombosis, which is a clot in these vessels instead of a mere narrowing, usually causes withering of a portion of heart muscle, which is replaced by scar tissue. During this phase of the disease, bed rest and other treatment are essential. The size of the scar, termed a healed myocardial infarction, determines the degree of impairment of cardiac reserve. If the scar is small, the change in the function of the pump may be undetectable.

d) Arteriosclerotic heart disease. Arteriosclerotic heart disease causes a diffuse, usually microscopic, scarring in the heart muscle that mechanically interferes with its contraction. This disorder leads to various disturbances of heart rhythm which decrease its efficiency, comparable to what happens in an automobile motor whose timer is not functioning properly. The most frequent of these disturbances of rhythm, extrasystoles or premature contractions, are scarcely ever of clinical significance.

e) Hypertensive heart disease or high blood pressure. Several varieties of high blood pressure have been determined, but the most frequently encountered type merely intensifies the work of the heart by the increase in the pressure part of the engineer's formula previously given. Waste is not apparent in the output factor as in the case of congenital or rheumatic heart disease, and defects do not occur in the heart muscle at least for many years.

ACTIVITIES OF THE PATIENT WITH CHRONIC HEART DISEASE

In general, the patient with chronic heart disease does best if he lives so that he uses some or much of his cardiac reserve almost every day. Heart reserve is not like financial reserve in that it tends to increase with use if it is never pushed to the point of exhaustion. A patient with chronic heart disease should be able to control his ac-

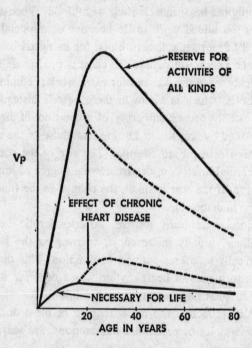

Cardiac reserve, or the ability of the heart to respond to increased demands for energy, is illustrated in this schematic graph. Since the heart is essentially a pump, its work can be expressed in mechanical terms: work = Vp (volume or output of fluid, i.e., blood, multiplied by the amount of pressure). The minimum and maximum levels of work that the heart can do are indicated by the two solid curved lines. The effects of chronic heart disease are represented by the dotted lines, which indicate the increase in the minimum necessary to maintain life and the decided decrease in the maximum. The heart of a healthy individual in his twenties can do more than twenty times the work per minute for short intervals than is required simply to keep him alive.

tivities and stop them temporarily, frequently momentarily, if he has symptoms which warn him that he is approaching his limits.

These limits vary from person to person, from the restrictions that ordinarily apply to people without heart disease to those that require a severe change in the *modus operandi*. The patient whose activities need not be restricted may lead a normal life without any heart consciousness. His only problems will relate to military, insurance, and pre-employment physical examinations. Those persons with known organic heart disease should learn what symptoms to heed in their particular cases. The great majority of these patients lead active, useful lives for many years.

Several symptoms can serve as warnings that patients may be exceeding their speed limits. Some of them are common to most all forms of heart ailments and some apply more to specific diseases. They will be described separately:

a) Shortness of breath (dyspnea). An increase in the rate and depth of breathing occurs when we are physically active. If we halt what we are doing, this agitation should calm down in a short time, about one minute, unless the activity has been excessive. The patient with known heart disease should yield relatively early to this shortness of breath. If it subsides promptly, he may resume the activity that caused it, preferably at a slower pace. If it persists for several minutes or longer, he should not attempt to repeat that task that day and not at the same rate in the future. If it continues for an hour or more, medical help is advisable and essential.

b) Pain in the chest (coronary pain). Typically, coronary pain is underneath the breast bone and may travel to one or both arms or the neck. The patient should submit to it as soon as he becomes aware that an attack is beginning and not wait even the seconds that are usually required for the pain to increase in severity to the point where it makes him stop. Often these coronary pains arise as a result of a combination of two or more circumstances, each of which requires increased work of the heart. The businessman who takes a client to lunch, discusses an important project, walks back to the office on a cold, windy day up a little hill or ramp is more likely to get this pain in his chest, if he has the foundation for it, than if he abstained from doing some of these things simultaneously. A variant of this type of pain may awaken the patient in the early morning. Usually he will be more comfortable sooner if he sits up in bed or even in a chair. If the pain persists for more than half an hour, it is advisable to summon a physician.

c) Excessive fatigue. All of us get tired occasionally, particularly at the end of the day. The heart patient who notices that he is becoming fatigued more frequently and earlier in the day should take stock of his activities and endeavor to curtail them. A classical example of such a situation arises when a young woman with rheumatic heart disease has multiple pregnancies and no help with the major household jobs. Even with modern appliances some of these tasks are peculiarly tiring. Some, which have not changed much, such as washing walls, windows, and floors and making beds, are among the most trying for her. This young woman may notice chronic fatigue before she is aware of any shortness of breath while performing these chores. It would seem advisable and wiser to employ a cleaning woman, if one can be obtained, than to risk slipping into congestive heart failure.

d) Swelling of the ankles. In the summertime, many people, especially obese women, have some swelling of the ankles at the end of the day. Those with known heart disease may find this symptom, like fatigue, a timely signal that they are doing too much.

e) Pain below the right rib margin. Pain in the upper right side of the abdomen on exertion may be the best warning for a few patients. It may be felt before any awareness of shortness of breath is noted. Such pain is caused by a sudden congestion and swelling of the liver when the cardiac reserve has been exceeded. Usually it does not subside as quickly as shortness of breath does when the activity is stopped, and therefore such discomfort should be taken seriously. It should be regarded, together with fatigue and swelling of the ankles, as evidence that the over-all way of life is too strenuous.

f) Loss of appetite. Loss of appetite, sometimes accompanied by actual nausea, is a symptom relative in significance to that of pain in the upper right side of the abdomen. It presents a problem to the physician because it must be distinguished from the side-effects of some of the drugs that are prescribed to bolster the circulation. Simple restriction of activity for a few days can often alleviate such loss of appetite without medication.

g) Pounding of the heart (palpitation). Awareness of palpitation, or pounding of the heart, of forceful, sometimes rapid heartbeats, is only rarely useful as a symptom to patients. In general, they should avoid cultivating a particular interest in their heart's action. Those who do have disturbances of heart rhythm at times should take cognizance of such palpitation.

h) Congestive heart failure. Congestive heart failure is a derangement of the circulation in which one or all of the already discussed symptoms, together with various findings on physical examination, are persistent in spite of severely restricted activity. This heart failure requires complete bed rest. Modern medication has so improved such conditions and the outlook for these patients that many of them can return to full-time work when the episode has passed.

CONCLUSION

The patient with organic heart disease should be as active as he can be without producing harm. Many can lead essentially normal lives. Those who require rest would do well to learn and know their special warnings of when they are approaching the limits of their cardiac reserve. These signals are more important to them than any arbitrary regimen of so many flights of stairs, blocks of walking, and other quotas. Emotional stresses increase the work of the heart and sometimes are the only factors that elicit these warnings. Such patients should endeavor to regulate their lives so that they are in control of their activities at all times. This may require changes which vary in severity from relinquishing a job which demands excessive physical work to foregoing the pleasures of watching a wrestling match on television.

NOTES ON THE CONTRIBUTING SPECIALISTS

EMMET B. BAY is professor of medicine at the University of Chicago Medical School. He was born in Illinois in 1901 and received his degree in medicine from Rush Medical College, Chicago, in 1923.

THOMAS J. DRY, now in private practice in Cape Town, in his native South Africa, was until recently professor of medicine at the University of Minnesota, and at the Mayo Clinic. After receiving degrees in medicine and surgery at the University of Cape Town, he came to the United States to study at the University of Minnesota, and was a Fellow of the Mayo Foundation before joining the staff of the University.

MORRIS FISHBEIN is the author or editor of numerous books of medical information for the layman, and is medical editor of the *Britannica Book of the Year*. For more than thirty-five years, he was with the American Medical Association. Dr. Fishbein was born in St. Louis, Missouri, and received his degree in medicine from Rush Medical College, Chicago, in 1912.

GEORGE R. HERRMANN is professor of medicine at the University of Texas. He was born in Indiana and received his degree in medicine from the University of Michigan in 1918.

REXFORD KENNAMER is clinic physician at Cedars of Lebanon Hospital in Beverly Hills, California, where he is associated with Dr. Myron Prinzmetal. He was born in Alabama and received his degree in medicine from Jefferson Medical College, Philadelphia, in 1945.

ANCEL KEYS is director of the laboratory of physiological hygiene at the University of Minnesota School of Public Health and expert consultant to the United Nations' Food and Agriculture Organization and World Health Organization. He was born in Colorado and received his Ph.D. in physiology from the University of California in 1930. With his wife, he is the author of a popular book on diet and health, *Eat Well and Stay Well*.

RICHARD P. LASSER is assistant attending cardiologist at Mount Sinai Hospital, New York, where he is associated with Dr. Arthur Master. He was born in New York and received his degree in medicine from the College of Physicians and Surgeons, Columbia University, New York, in 1945.

ALDO A. LUISADA is associate professor of medicine at Chicago Medical College and attending cardiologist at Mt. Sinai Hospital, Chicago. He is editor of a system of cardiology sponsored by the American College of Cardiology. He was graduated in 1925 from the Medical School of the University of Florence, Italy.

ARTHUR M. MASTER is chief of the cardiography laboratory and cardiac clinics at Mount Sinai Hospital, New York. He was born in New York and received his degree in medicine from Cornell University in 1921. During the War, Dr. Master was a captain in the Naval Reserve and chief of medicine at U.S. Mobile Hospital No. 10, in the Solomon Islands. He is the author of some 280 articles on cardiac diseases.

IRVINE H. PAGE is director of the research division of the Cleveland (Ohio) Clinic Foundation. He was born in Indiana and received his degree in medicine from Cornell University in 1921. Before going to the Cleveland Clinic, he was associated with the Rockefeller Institute for Medical Research, New York. He is a former president of the American Heart Association.

WILLIS J. POTTS is surgeon-in-chief at Children's Memorial Hospital, Chicago, and professor of pediatric surgery at Northwestern University. He was born in Wisconsin and received his degree in medicine from Rush Medical College, Chicago, in 1923.

WALTER S. PRIEST is attending physician at Wesley Memorial Hospital, Chicago, consulting internist at St. Francis Hospital, Evanston, and professor of medicine at Northwestern University. He was born in Colorado and received his degree in medicine from Washington University, St. Louis, in 1920.

MYRON PRINZMETAL is chief cardiologist at City of Hope, Los Angeles, attending physician at Cedars of Lebanon Hospital, Beverly Hills, and associate clinical professor of medicine at the University of California at Los Angeles. He was born in New York and received his degree in medicine from the University of California in 1933.

NORMAN B. ROBERG is attending physician at Illinois Research and Education Hospital and associate professor of medicine at the University of Illinois. He was born in Chicago and received his degree in medicine from Harvard University in 1934.

DAVID SCHERF is attending physician at Flower-Fifth Avenue Hospital, New York, and professor of clinical medicine at New York Medical College. He was born in Austria and received his degree in medicine from the University of Vienna in 1922.

ISAAC STARR has been Hartzell Professor of therapeutics research at the University of Pennsylvania since 1933, with an interval as dean of the University's Medical School, 1945–48. He was born in Philadelphia and received his degree in medicine from the University of Pennsylvania in 1920.

GENE H. STOLLERMAN is consulting cardiologist at Children's Memorial Hospital, Chicago, and associate professor of medicine at Northwestern University. He was born in New York and received his degree in medicine at the College of Physicians and Surgeons, Columbia University, in 1944.

MORRIS W. STROUD III is associate director of medical service at Highland View Hospital, Cleveland, and associate professor of medicine at Western Reserve University. He was born in Pennsylvania and received his degree in medicine from the University of Pennsylvania in 1939.

EDWARD WEISS (1895–1960) was attending physician at Temple University Hospital, Philadelphia, and professor of clinical medicine at Temple University. He was born in Pennsylvania and received his degree in medicine from Jefferson Medical College, Philadelphia, in 1917.

PAUL DUDLEY WHITE is a noted consultant on cardiac diseases. From 1920 to 1949 he was chief of cardiac clinics and laboratories at Massachusetts General Hospital, Boston. At present he is consultant in medicine at Massachusetts General and professor of clinical medicine at Harvard University. He was born in Boston and received his degree in medicine from Harvard in 1911.

INDEX